FATAL TO FEARLESS

FATAL TO FEAR*LESS*

12 Steps to Beating Cancer in a Broken Medical System

Kathy Giusti

HARPER WAVE
An Imprint of HarperCollins*Publishers*

HarperCollins books may be purchased for educational, business, or sales promotional use. For information, please email the Special Markets Department at SPsales@harpercollins.com.

FIRST EDITION

Designed by Bonni Leon-Berman

Library of Congress Cataloging-in-Publication Data has been applied for.

ISBN 978-0-06-328217-9

24 25 26 27 28 LBC 6 5 4 3 2

To FamJam,

I love you.

CONTENTS

Foreword by Katie Couric

We've all known people in our lives who have made lemonade out of lemons. That's what Kathy Giusti did when she was diagnosed with multiple myeloma, a rare blood cancer. Kathy not only cured herself, but she created a whole lemonade factory that has helped hundreds of thousands of people who have been diagnosed with cancer.

I first met Kathy at a memorial service in Connecticut for David Bloom, an NBC reporter and anchor who had died of a pulmonary embolism while covering the war in Iraq. David was young, vibrant, a terrific correspondent with a beautiful family. It was hard to believe that his life had been cut tragically short when he was just thirty-nine.

When Kathy introduced herself, I had no idea that it would be the beginning of what would become a lifetime connection. She wanted to thank me for all the work I'd done to raise awareness for cancer. But the more we talked, and the more I heard her story, I quickly realized we had something else in common. Kathy knew what it felt like to be diagnosed with a terminal illness for which there was no cure.

I knew that feeling all too well, watching two people I loved go through the same thing. I lost my husband Jay to stage four colon cancer in 1998. He was forty-two. My sister Emily died of pancreatic cancer a few years later at fifty-four. Kathy had been told she had three years to live in 1996. She was thirty-seven. There was nothing she could do—there was no treatment, no drugs, not even experimental ones. In other words, the kind of punch-you-in-the-gut, this-can't-be-happening life-shattering news that you can't even wrap your brain around. But here she was, six years later, emanating vibrancy, determination, and very much alive. I wondered, who was this cancer-fighting superhero? And how did she do this?

First, Kathy had the tools in her toolkit to change the paradigm and potentially cure an uncurable cancer. As a rising business executive at a leading pharmaceutical company, she had an inside view into the healthcare system—how research was conducted, how drugs were developed, and how they ultimately found their way to patients. Then, as a patient, she had a front-row seat to that same healthcare system. Facing mountains of red tape, hours on hold, and the all-too-often repeated "I'd like to help you, but . . ." Kathy refused to take no for an answer. In the end, she not only saved her own life, but disrupted a deeply broken healthcare system in ways that would help millions of others facing a fatal diagnosis.

But while Kathy became a badass, ball-busting, cancer-fighting whiz, she never lost her humanity. She has helped countless people navigate their way from diagnosis to treatment, often serving as a one-woman clearinghouse of invaluable advice and life-saving information. Friend or colleague, celebrity or stranger, when a cancer patient called, Kathy always answered. One such patient was my friend Eliza's father. Eliza was a member of our staff at KCM, the media company my husband and I started. When her father was diagnosed, Kathy got on the phone with Eliza's dad right away, put together a team, connected him with a doctor at Dana Farber, made sure he was getting the tests he needed and got him the best care possible. For Eliza, who was only in her twenties and not prepared to be a caregiver, Kathy was a much-needed lifesaver. When another dear friend, Mimi, was diagnosed with a very tough myeloma, Kathy showed her the power of following the research. She helped her get her genome sequenced then moved her from one cutting-edge treatment to the next, from transplant to a precision medicine designed for her specific cancer, to a breakthrough CAR-T cell therapy which is keeping her cancer at bay.

Sadly, we can't clone Kathy—but this book is the next best thing. A road map for every patient who hears those three words: you have cancer. When my husband and sister were diagnosed, I remember being in a complete mental fog, lost and afraid and not knowing where to turn for real, practical advice. How do you know how to get to the right doctors? What is the best treatment? Does my insurance cover it? Is there a clinical trial and should I be in it? After years of coaching patients, navigating medical centers, biomarker tests, genomic tests, immune tests, Kathy knows what to do. She has identified simple and actionable steps any patient can take to access the best care available. Given the extraordinary speed of today's scientific advancements, that additional year, or two, or three, can get you a lifetime.

Kathy's is a deeply personal story that has had a profound public impact. Now we can all be the beneficiaries of her experience and wisdom that comes from the most motivating of all conditions—the desire to live. When *Time* magazine asked me to write about Kathy for their list of 100 Most Influential People issue in 2011, it was a tremendous honor. I called her a hero then. She's still a hero to me. And after reading this book, hearing her kind, compassionate voice girded with steely determination tell you her story, she will be your hero too—and a much-needed companion as you or someone you love faces a challenging diagnosis.

—Katie Couric

Introduction

If today you were given a scant three years (or less) to live, what would you do? When I was given a fatal cancer diagnosis more than twenty-five years ago, I was told that's how long I had. Back then, I was a rising pharmaceutical executive who would have been a doctor had my physician father not urged me to stay on the business side. I knew the science and the industry, but I didn't know how challenging it would be to work the healthcare system until I found myself in it as a patient. In truth, I was scared shitless.

The road to my cure was not an easy one to walk, let alone run as fast as possible. I felt encumbered by a system that didn't have my death sentence in mind. A system that could take its time while mine was running out. It sparked a level of incalculable drive, forcing me to shift from fear to fearless if I was going to survive. Cancer does what cancer does—anything. And *despite* you. I had to grow a new spine, as it were, and learn a new dialect that may as well have been a foreign language. The experience ultimately launched me into the role of a lifetime as I turned a single "WTF" mortality (reality) check into the greatest lifeline. Between fighting for my own survival and decoding the complex system along the way, which took me to leadership roles at places like the National Cancer Institute (NCI) and my own research foundation, I figured out a recipe—a list of WTDs (what to do). It came in handy when, in 2022, I received a new diagnosis, this time breast cancer. My second round in the ring was not against a death sentence, thankfully, but it was equally as humbling and harrowing for its own reasons. I had to learn hard lessons over again, question everything, lean once more on family members and friends for help, surrender to the whims of such a wily disease in a yet-still-broken system, and find some new ingredients for my playbook to get through it. Indeed, when facing a terrifying diagnosis, even an expert needs help.

As happens with writing a book, the process took on a life of its own. Admittedly, I initially sought to write my "twelve-step formula" for finding cures like an instruction manual, letting those steps delineate and dominate the narrative. But truth be told, the journey I took was more complex. It was about fears and family, gambles and barters, prayers and apologies, feelings and frustrations, photos and ticket stubs, unspoken words, and relentless drive. A punishing drive—on me and everyone around me. The playbook to survival is ultimately about people. As I lived past those three years and kept going, catching glimmers of hope for more time and dashing toward them, I only grew more dogged, more fearless. And that fearlessness was on behalf of everyone seeking a path to a cure.

In writing this book, I went back to the journals I'd kept every year through my survival—twenty-five now and counting, chronicling a life for decades in different-sized and -colored volumes, each hand chosen by a family member or friend. Inside were my most personal notes, sometimes scribbled quickly, sometimes bulleted, sometimes deep and thoughtful. They were at times joyous, other times not easy to read. Reading between the lines, I knew when I was happy, mad, hopeful, scared, grateful, sorry, or desperate. Within the pages were the written clues to how my life greatly impacted those around me. Some of my greatest gifts, like being daring and determined to win over my disease, became my greatest curses in many ways. Of course, there are costs that come with illness, costs you'll read about in these pages, and which became astonishingly clear to me as I wrote the book.

Although my story is one of cancer, what I learned applies to anyone going through an illness. I've worn all the shoes, both as a patient, a caregiver, and a leader driving change within the healthcare system. I've watched people I care about go through so much suffering. And I want you to know what I've learned so you can benefit. I care so damn much about patients and their families. We all deserve a fighting chance no matter what. Perhaps nothing is more humanizing than a dance with death.

Everyone is touched by a serious and scary diagnosis at some point, be it their own or that of a loved one. But not everyone has access to the right information and direction, or simply the know-how to gain that access. Until now. On the other side of the bad news— "You have [fill in the disease]"—is the good news: Getting diagnosed today is not like it was two decades ago, or even a few years ago. Sure, there's still a lot of fear and unknowns (and no guaranteed remedies for many ills), but the hope for a longer, fulfilling life is exponentially greater—and possible. Today, if you don't know what to do, you have much more to lose.

One of the first people I reached out to when writing this book was Eric Topol. He is among the most brilliant minds in scientific circles today and an outspoken champion for change. He is also one of the most patient-focused physicians I know. I remember our traveling together when we were on the same advisory board years ago, and I've always been blown away by his sense of empathy toward patients. Our conversations were always the same: how fast science and technology are moving, how slowly the system is changing to catch up. That's why Eric wrote his 2015 book *The Patient Will See You Now*, which describes a "Gutenberg moment" where people are largely in charge of their healthcare thanks to technology. Eric truly wanted to shift the power to the patient. But in talking with Eric today, he has yet to see that moment. "I haven't seen much change," he admits with disappointment. The system continues to fall behind the speed of science, leaving patients uninformed and on their own.

My next conversation was with Clifford Hudis, CEO of the American Society of Clinical Oncology (ASCO). He echoed Topol's frustrations. More than half of people don't understand basic aspects of the healthcare system, and when you bring a forbidding diagnosis into the fold of such healthcare illiteracy, you can imagine the trouble that looms and what's at stake (a life). The system is deplorably fragmented, bureaucratic, and exceedingly complex, shaped by many different needs and incentives, and it does not play to benefit you and me, who are left wasting time trying to work the system. Clifford put the status quo quite bluntly: "We do not have a system in the US. No strategic plan for healthcare. No mission statements. No set of goals. No national agenda. And you can quote me on that: We do not have a system. Full stop."

But despite what at times can feel like a full systemic breakdown, both Topol and Hudis still have hope. We all agreed I needed to write this book because in the end, the power is in us, the patient. And we can be inspired to lead ourselves and generate our own personal methods for making "the system" work for each and every one of us. No matter how fearful we are of our diagnosis, we can find a way to beat the system, to turn the volume down on our fear—to fear *less*. The key is to approach a diagnosis in a systematic fashion, act quickly, and continually figure it out as you go just like I did (and still do!). And only then will the system become more accessible and friendlier, and help us all. Patients often become not only active disease advocates but also active researchers to change the healthcare system.

The book is organized around twelve steps but is also flanked by an intimate narrative that speaks to the greater, often unspeakable challenges of dealing with sickness. Each chapter takes one step in turn with clear and specific WTDs outlined and includes input from experts I've interviewed to round out conversations. In Part 1, the first four steps take you through the motions of nailing your diagnosis, learning the landscape of your disease, and preparing for treatment with both personal and medical goals in mind. Then, Part 2 guides you through the treatment process with plenty of extra advice to deal with unexpected setbacks, including recurrences. Part 3 shows you how to stay on top of the science, actively live in prevention mode, and thrive. And the epilogue ties the book together with final revelations on some of the hardest lessons I've learned, and codas to the storytelling. While this all sounds methodical and straightforward, the journey is anything but. After all, this is about life. And life is about relationships. May you find helpful tools and courage in these pages. Tools to strike the balance of living your life while saving your life. Tools to help you live *more* and fear *less*.

PART 1

The Wake-Up Call

Step 1

Understand the Diagnosis

Where Do I Start?

It begins with something. A wonky test result. A spot on an image. A surprising remark from your doctor on an otherwise regular visit—*there's one thing I'd like to check again . . . I don't understand . . . something is off . . . we need to take a closer look . . .*

The moment is vague, unsettling, an abrupt deviation from normal that sticks and you cannot unstick it. Whatever characterizes the moment, it's inescapable. You hold on to the notion that it could be nothing, but everything going forward feels a little unscripted, uncertain, and perhaps unbearable.

One in two people will develop cancer in their lifetime. If that happens to you or a loved one, there's no need to panic. Your first step should be to take a deep breath. Your body senses your fear; it might go into flight, fight, or freeze mode. But stop and focus. Take your time. Now, you're most likely going to head to your smartphone or computer. That's fine. The vast majority of people diagnosed with cancer, 89 percent according to one survey, search online to get answers.* Step 1 helps you do it right, quietly and methodically, so you find the best information for your situation.

---

*   This figure is based on a Healthline-commissioned survey from 2017. It is cited by Ann Meredith Garcia Trinidad in her article for Cancer.net. See: "How to Tell If Cancer Information on Social Media Is 'Fake News'" (September 29, 2020).

Christmas, 1995

It was a mere four days before Christmas. My husband, Paul, and I had decorated our first Christmas tree in our new home, the one we'd both worked so hard to buy. Our eighteen-month-old daughter, Nicole, had been fascinated by the glint of the tinsel and the stuffed Rudolph she'd found in one of the boxes. After we put her to bed, Paul and I celebrated with a glass of wine, a rare treat on a weekday night given our schedules.

"Look how far we've come together," I said, resting my head on Paul's shoulder. "I love seeing Christmas through Nicole's eyes." As I spoke the words, I could hear my biological clock ticking through the Christmas album playing on low volume in the background.

I'd been feeling uncharacteristically run-down at thirty-seven years old and was having trouble conceiving our second child. I'd also unintentionally lost a little weight, which I chalked up to a recent business trip abroad that wore me out. Paul and I were mentally preparing for fertility treatments, perhaps IVF, and I had an appointment with my internist, Dr. Donald Steinmuller, the next morning for some tests. Before seeing a fertility specialist, my primary care doctor had to do some blood work on me for insurance purposes. I rushed to get the tests done before the holiday break so I could start the new year with new hope. My job was chaotic at the best of times, and I was so ecstatic to have the week off between Christmas and New Year's with Paul and Nicole that I didn't think twice when Steinmuller asked me to repeat the tests after Christmas.

The first week of January had me immediately back to work—three days onstage at a big regional sales meeting I was leading in downtown Chicago. As the executive director of Midwest operations for Searle's fleet of drugs, I was on track to become a high-level senior executive at the company, handpicked by my mentor Al Heller, who also happened to be Searle's chief operating officer (COO). I was being pushed outside my comfort zone with each rotation I was asked to take. My background was strategy and marketing; now I was in charge of educating, motivating, and training our sales force to build the company's presence in hospitals and doctors' offices.

After being "on" for three straight days, I returned home to a cryptic note Paul had left on the counter in his scribbled handwriting. It read *hemoglobin low, hematocrit low, protein high*. I didn't know what that meant for us. Was it just about my attempts to get pregnant? At the bottom of the note: "see us together." A clear sign something was wrong. Doctors didn't tell patients to come in with their spouses unless something was horribly awry. That much I knew from being the daughter of a physician.

"Paul, I'm really worried—this is bad," I had said reflexively. "How long has this been sitting here? When did the doctor call? How did he sound?"

I knew that routine test results could be given over the phone, but something didn't feel right. Paul had assured me the doctor sounded "fine" and merely wanted to "look at a few things." Now I was awaiting a callback that would change the course of my life. That call didn't come in until I was speeding along the Edens Expressway during evening rush hour. His sense of urgency was not lost on me.

"Can you and Paul come in tomorrow?" Steinmuller asked. "I know it's Saturday, but I'll open up my office for you."

"So, what is it? What do you think I have?" I asked.

He hesitated again, as if fumbling for the right words. He again talked about abnormalities in my blood work. He said I was anemic. He recited what I'd read on the scribbled memo the night before. I pushed for more specifics and asked what an elevated protein indicated. He wasn't sure, and suggested I see a hematologist, a doctor who specialized in blood. Looking back now, I'm pretty sure he intentionally avoided telling me that blood doctors often doubled as oncologists—cancer doctors, or in the specific case of blood cancer doctors, "heme-oncs."

"You must have some suspicions," I probed. "What do you think

I have? Dr. Steinmuller, I'm not getting off this phone until I have a thought on what this might be."

"Okay, are you still driving?"

"Yes, but I'm fine. Just say it. Just tell me."

The doctor seemed to suppress what he was going to say next in a long pause, then finally let it out.

"I think you have multiple myeloma—but Kathy, we have to confirm it."

"I have no idea what that is," I said, slightly concussed and unable to understand him. I barely heard him telling me that many more tests needed to be performed.

"I can go over it all with you and Paul tomorrow morning," he said.

"What is that?" I asked.

"Well, you have cancer. It's a cancer of the bone marrow," he clarified, "a cancer of the plasma cells in your immune system."

And there it was—the first time I heard the C-word.

"How bad is it? How long do I have?" I asked in a surprisingly even tone.

"Let's not go there. We don't know what you have yet. It's premature. See me at eleven tomorrow. I can answer everything then."

It's hard not to panic when you're told you have cancer. It was just three years previously when my mom called to tell me about my father. Late-stage renal cell carcinoma. He should have seen the signs; it's not like you can miss blood in your urine. He was a doctor, after all—I guess even doctors don't like to face their own mortality. By the time they found my father's cancer, it was too late. Nine months later, he was gone. How could I not be scared?

That next morning, Paul, baby Nicole, and I set out to learn more. We camped out in the parking lot of a Borders at 9:45 a.m., fifteen minutes before it opened. It was our version of Google at the time. When the doors unlocked, I dashed through the store to the medical section, picked up the classic *Harrison's Internal Medicine*, and plunked myself down on the floor hoping to learn about multiple myeloma. Paul quickly leafed through the thick *Merck Manual* I handed him, checking the index first. We had less than an hour to figure this out. We planned to be ready with questions before our eleven o'clock appointment. We knew we were in for surprises and a steep learning curve, but we wanted a head start.

The tomes said little about my disease other than the fact it was a silent cancer of the bone marrow and there was no cure. Now I knew the meaning of a low reading of hemoglobin in my blood and a high measure of total protein. I also understood how unlikely it was for a young woman to develop this disease. I was an anomaly, and probably a soon-to-be-dead one. The knot in my stomach intensified and I broke into a cold sweat. I kept reading to secure something hopeful. Anything other than "fatal, treated with melphalan, leads to bone damage and kidney damage" and "depending on staging, patients live about three years." The chance of beating the disease altogether was zero.

There it was: I would not make it to my fortieth birthday, nor would I be there for our daughter's first day of kindergarten. My eyes latched on to the words "it can be found earlier in an MGUS or smoldering stage," whatever that meant. "It can be found as a single plasmacytoma completely radiated," whatever *that* meant. *Okay, maybe that's me? Please let that be me. Please don't tell me it's too late and I didn't catch this sooner when it was curable.*

The First To-Dos

There was no internet like today when I was first diagnosed with multiple myeloma. It was perfectly reasonable back then to wait for the local bookstore to open at ten a.m. on a Saturday and race to the medical section. Thank goodness I was already familiar with the medical lingo and could scan the information quickly to prepare for my appointment. I was crushed by the lack of information (and hope) in the textbooks. I knew we would have to do more research on our own. Lots of phone calls, the old-school way.

It would be a week before Christmas, nearly twenty-five years later, when I would face another cancer diagnosis. This time, breast cancer. And I still hear the words tumbling out of my doctor's mouth after my bi-annual screening: "We saw something . . . A spot . . . Could be nothing . . . Let's not take any chances . . . We should go in and check it out . . ."

It was déjà vu.

After I left her office, before even undergoing a biopsy, I did what everyone does today: I googled "early-stage breast cancer."

Nearly a billion results shot back on my smartphone. All I could think of was *WTF?!*

The Age of Information should be empowering. It should help us stay rational, calm, and fact-based. But what I encountered only made my head spin, ultimately disempowering me. I pressed pause, centered myself with a long, deep breath to slow my brain down, and shifted gears from WTF to WTD—What to Do to follow the rules I'd long learned the hard way.

STEP 1: UNDERSTAND THE DIAGNOSIS

WTDs

Search Wisely

X Be specific with your search words

X Know the different URLs

X Start with the leading sites

X Find disease-specific .orgs for your specific needs

X Look out for ads and expiration dates

X Follow the medical meetings

Phone, Subscribe, and Follow

X Start calling

X Sign up and subscribe

X Follow on social media

Use Your Portal

X Get logged in

X Know what to look for

WTD 1: Search Wisely

✓ *Be specific with your search words*

Whether it's Google, Bing, or the latest generative AI, the words you input matter. Put simply, how you tell the internet what you're seeking revolves around which words you choose, and the results you receive will be different based on those words. Searching for "skin cancer" will return different sites than if you had punched in "melanoma." Similarly, typing in "localized prostate cancer" will return results much different from "metastasized prostate cancer." The more precise you can be to your specific condition, the smarter your online hunting will be, and the more likely you are to obtain information that's relevant to you. Use words that your doctor said to you. And if you don't remember or are unsure, don't hesitate to call your doctor's office for clarification and to ask about more specifics relevant to you. Here are five simple search rules to help guide you toward the results you're looking for:

→ Words that state where *you* are in your journey: such as "newly diagnosed," "waiting results," "starting treatment"

→ Words that state where *your disease* is in its journey: "stage 1," "stage 2" . . .

→ Words that state your *specific disease*: not "skin cancer," but "melanoma" or "squamous cell"

→ Words that state your *specific type* of disease if you know it:

not just "breast cancer," but "estrogen receptor positive," "triple-negative," "HER-2," and "BRCA," etc.

→ Words that state your *specific needs*: "Questions to ask my doctor"

✓ *Know the different URLs*

Looking at the website root address or "unique resource locator" (URL) will quickly tell you what you might expect. When looking for health information, the most common root URLs end with one of the following:

→ .org (nonprofit organizations such as patient advocacy groups)

→ .edu (accredited academic centers)

→ .gov (government agencies such as the National Cancer Institute)

→ .com (diagnostic, pharma, and other health services companies)

While there's value to be found in all types of sites, it's good to begin with the ones noted below.

✓ *Start with the leading sites*

→ **Cancer.org**: The American Cancer Society (ACS) is the chief patient advocacy organization to provide high-quality content for patients and caregivers no matter what cancer you've been diagnosed with. The ACS's site (www.cancer.org) gets more than 50 million unique visitors a year and is cross-wired with Cancer.net. Together, this is your top resource to start.

→ **Cancer.net**: This is the American Society of Clinical Oncology's hub for people with cancer and their families. (Don't be fooled by the ".net"—the ACS already owned cancer.org.) Although ASCO is geared more toward clinicians, their patient-centric site at Cancer.net is designed to speak to everyone. These sites, in fact, share a lot in common and you'll find parallels and echoes in the information presented.

→ **Cancer.gov**: While not a .org, the National Cancer Institute (NCI) at www.Cancer.gov is the federal government's principal agency for cancer research and training and has some of the best information out there. The information is robust thanks to the National Cancer Institute's (NCI's) funding to many centers around the country.

→ **Mayoclinic.org**: The patient-friendly resource provided by the well-respected Mayo Clinic.

✓ *Find disease-specific .orgs for your specific needs*

While the broader .orgs give you a great foundation, you will also find that there are disease-specific .orgs that are tailored to speak to your specific disease. They will often come up immediately as a .org in your original search. If you don't see one, try searching for an "advocacy group or research foundation" in your cancer. Once you find one, be sure to look at the "About Us" section. It will share the group's mission, programming, executive team, even financials. You want to work with a group that is accredited by Charity Navigator (CharityNavigator.org), which lists financial accreditations of various charities on its website. Some excellent examples include:

→ Breastcancer.org

→ FightColorectalCancer.org

→ The Leukemia and Lymphoma Society at www.lls.org

→ LUNGevity Foundation at www.lungevity.org

→ Multiple Myeloma Research Foundation at www.themmrf.org

→ Pancreatic Cancer Action Network at www.pancan.org

→ The Prostate Cancer Foundation at www.pcf.org

→ Susan G. Komen at www.komen.org

✓ *Look out for ads and expiration dates*

There are a few things to look out for as you search wisely. To help spot sites with hidden agendas, look for links tagged as "Ad"— especially those close to the top of your main search page. The information may be excellent, but the "ad" means they are paying to drive you to that site. It may be because they want you to call a specific medical center or be aware of a specific drug for your cancer. The information may be valid, but in early searches, you want to start with agenda-free information regarding where to go and what to take.

Also be sure to check the date. Not all information has an expiration date, but with science moving at increasing speed, you don't want to make health decisions based on outdated information. Credible sites will list dates when material was published. If not found on top of the article, check the bottom of the page or within the URL for a date. You want material that's been updated within the last one to three years if possible. Much depends on how much progress is being made in that cancer at the time.

✓ *Follow the medical meetings*

It's also good to track the key medical meetings for the latest news related to your specific cancer. Most significant are the annual meetings for the American Society of Clinical Oncology (ASCO) and the American Association for Cancer Research (AACR), which feature research across all cancers, and the American Society of Hematology (ASH), which focuses on blood cancers. There are also meetings focused on specific cancers such as the San Antonio Breast Cancer Symposium (SABCS). All of these meetings present cutting-edge research findings and clinical trial results and are worth following on their social media channels. (For more info on these meetings, see Step 7 on getting the right treatment.)

WTD 2: Phone, Subscribe, and Follow

✓ *Start calling*

Once you've identified the organizations for you, call their 800 numbers and helplines to ask what specific resources they offer beyond their website. Questions to ask include:

→ Do you offer physician referrals?

→ Do you have any upcoming educational programs?

→ Do you have patient navigators? Are they trained nurses? Do you have patient mentors who have been through my experience?

✓ *Sign up and subscribe*

Sites will often ask you to sign up for more information. This is worth doing. If you don't sign up or register, you will not receive the current information these organizations offer. Provide your email or other contact information to receive newsletters, join virtual events, chats, and webinars. The information is almost always free of charge and highly informative. You can also ask your family to register as well.

✓ *Follow your top sites on social media*

As you do your searches, look out for organizations you want to follow. Most of them will have Facebook and Instagram pages, which are an easy way to keep up with their latest news and events and start feeling a sense of community. If you're not a social media person, set up Google alerts by organization name or by type of cancer. You may also come across key opinion leaders (KOLs), leading doctors in the space, who share the most recent scientific and drug development information on social media. Follow them on Twitter, LinkedIn, or other channels.

WTD 3: Use Your Portal

✓ *Get logged in*

Your patient portal is a secure online website that gives you access to your personal health information from anywhere with an internet connection. Just as you do online banking and manage your money with a secure website or "financial portal," you use a patient portal to help manage your healthcare and keep track of doctor visits, test results, prescriptions, billing, etc. (see below). You will get information on the portal when you visit the doctor's office. If you need help setting it up with a username and password, ask the front desk to help you that day. And store your password somewhere where you won't lose it. Today, an increasing number of patients are using at least one portal but many still do not, partly because they don't know how to get on. It's absolutely worth your time.

✓ *Know what to look for*

Your portal will become your gateway to knowing everything about your disease. It is going to give you important benefits and empower you on the journey:

→ **Test results**: Access to lab results and radiology reports—both current and historical

→ **Secure messaging**: An efficient way to communicate with your doctor and nurses

→ **Appointments**: Efficiently schedule or reschedule appointments

→ **Medicines**: Access full medication lists, as well as request refills

→ **Billing and payments**: Access to your billing statements, payment history, and ability to make online payments

→ **Educational resources**: Healthcare providers often include valuable resources to help you understand your health status or treatment

IN CONVERSATION WITH KAREN KNUDSEN

Chief Executive Officer of the American Cancer Society

Karen E. Knudsen, MBA, PhD, came to the American Cancer Society (ACS) with an extraordinary medical background and a mission to elevate cancer patients' experience in their journey—from first diagnosis through survivorship. When you start searching online for information on cancer, chances are you'll come across her organization's site (Cancer.org) or its sister site at fightcancer.org run by ACS's advocacy affiliate, the American Cancer Society Cancer Action Network (ACS CAN). These are two of the best cancer sites for patients and families, reaching over 50 million unique visitors a year. I was excited to speak to her about her work and "best practices" for conducting prudent online searches.

Q. How can an organization like yours help patients?
A.   Since I began my job at the ACS, we've established a three-pillar model to improve the lives of cancer patients and their families: research, advocacy, and patient support. Everyone touched by cancer clamors for evidence-based guidance and information free of commercial influence and at a level they can understand. From my perspective, the key stakeholders are the patients and their families and caregivers. Communicating to them about how to navigate their care, and providing data-driven counsel backed by the highest-quality experts is a top goal. It's how we help empower patients and their families. When you're dealing with cancer, what you need is truth and a focus on how the field is changing. What is the most current information on coverage, treatment, and testing? ACS CAN is our nonprofit, nonpartisan

advocacy affiliate that works to influence critical public health policies important to our cancer mission, such as gaining additional access to healthcare coverage, and helps educate on how we can all get involved in creating a more equitable cancer journey. Another key element in our work is listening to and responding to patients. We don't have all the answers and welcome feedback to continually improve. The more we hear from patients, the better we can build and expand our resources and services and, ultimately, reduce cancer mortality.

Q. Cancer.org and Cancer.net are models for online destinations that feature cancer information. What should patients be looking for when conducting their searches?

A.   No matter where you go for information online upon a cancer diagnosis, you want to land on reliable sites and start in the right direction. This means finding unbiased information that's written, checked, and approved by medical professionals, and hopefully by those who are cancer experts. Check for credentials. It also helps if everything is organized in a way that's user-friendly to find what you're looking for, and it's revised and updated frequently. That's what we do at Cancer.org and what our friends and partners at the American Society of Clinical Oncology (ASCO) do at Cancer.net. ACS focuses on information tailored to the patients and families at Cancer.org, while ASCO's Cancer.net represents clinicians and educational content targeted to them. But we're not the only places to find information. When you're first diagnosed, it can be overwhelming to scroll through so much online, and sorting through what you need is time-consuming. As you move from one site to another, be aware of credibility. Check where the information is coming from, know who is behind it and why (e.g., who paid or sponsored the published information?), and be careful of sites composed of opinion and testimonials that are not grounded in science.

Q. Why should patients register or create accounts on sites?

A.   Many respectable sites for cancer information and resources have ways to engage and I highly recommend it, even if it means signing up with more than one site. We encourage patients to sign up on ours so they automatically receive emails to get the newest information and alerts about our ongoing programs and services, including information on how to get involved and volunteer. Family members and caregivers are also encouraged to sign up. Like many other sites, we have separate landing pages specifically designed for them so they know what to expect, what services can help them out, and what they need to know from day one. Also look for twenty-four/seven helplines that are staffed by trained cancer information specialists who can answer questions about a diagnosis and give guidance, including tips relevant to where you are geographically located. At Cancer.org, for example, we can connect patients and caregivers to others with similar experiences.

❋

"It's Myeloma."

"Are you sure this is what I have?" I asked, sitting in Dr. Steinmuller's office. I had just come from Borders, where I read that multiple myeloma was a disease that largely affected men, Black people, and the elderly.

"Kathy, I can't be positive until we do some scans and a bone marrow biopsy. Our next step is to get you to Dr. Slivnik." David Slivnik was the hematologist-oncologist (heme-onc, as they are called) at the local community hospital who would verify Steinmuller's hunch that I might have myeloma.

Dr. Slivnik was young, with a kind face and a direct nature. Time slowed to a grueling pace as he scheduled my bone marrow biopsy to confirm the disease and a series of full body scans to determine if it had started destroying my bones. It took time to fit me in and even more time to get the results. We were anxious and I kept staring at the kitchen phone waiting for him to call. Eventually it rang. The receptionist was on the other end asking us to come in. My fate would have to wait for Dr. Slivnik in person. We drove to the appointment with knots in our stomachs.

"Dr. Steinmuller was right," Slivnik said plainly. "You do have myeloma. The bone marrow biopsy confirmed it. But your scans don't show any lesions, which is a good thing."

"What exactly does that mean?" I asked. "I read that I only have three years. Is that true?"

"Let's take a deep breath," Dr. Slivnik said while resting a calming hand on my shoulder. "One thing at a time. We need to know more. Much more."

I barely recall the details of that conversation other than confirming I had cancer. A rare cancer with little in the pipeline to treat. Thrown into the cold, alienating, byzantine world of a grim diagnosis, my brain fired in all directions. How could I beat this? Where did I go wrong? Why was this happening? I would now live permanently in urgent mode. I kept myself together until Paul and I were in the parking lot. I sobbed in his arms, feeling a strong wave of unraveling. Then I insisted we return to the bookstore. We sat on the floor in the aisle with all the medical books splayed in front of us. We read every word about myeloma, took notes, and started to educate ourselves on potential treatments. There wasn't much. At this point, I only knew the name of my disease; I did not know my "stage" in the disease or what type or classification of multiple myeloma I had. Slivnik told me to be patient as I now went through the process—a process of diagnosing that would seem to take a thousand years.

Near the bookstore's exit, I grabbed a journal and new calendar that would lord over this new, marked period in our lives. My journal would log my thoughts and my day planner, which kept my work schedule straight, would be replaced by the calendar for endless doctor appointments, second opinions, and tests.

That night, Paul and I took the Christmas decorations down.

"Remember this one?" I said as I carefully wrapped a hand-painted glass ornament for what I thought might be the last time. "We got this on the day trip we took to Nantucket to celebrate the end of business school. You got so seasick on the ferry. We still had so much fun."

The tree was made up of memories, ornaments for every excursion we'd ever taken, magical freeze-frames of our life together I can still recall when I think about the "before" part—before cancer would draw a dividing line in our family. *I'm never going to open this box again*, I thought.

A huge chunk of me was still processing the fact that an innocent visit to the internist for a fertility referral had turned into a death sentence. With all the doctors' appointments, bookstore visits, and desperate attempts to learn more, learn *something*, I hadn't taken the time to sit down and let myself truly feel the emotions coursing through me. I was scared to leave. To leave Paul, to leave Nicole. I wondered what my life had meant. And with three years left, what would my life be?

Before going to bed, I sent an email to my office telling them I was sick and would miss a few more days. That was an understatement. At the back of my mind I was thinking everything I'd worked toward was done.

Then I did what I always do when I'm in a WTF moment. *Start with a blank piece of paper*, I told myself. A mantra for the many WTF moments I'd face going forward. I opened the journal I'd bought on the way out of Borders and started writing to Nicole. It was a small notebook with a yellow-orange sunflower on its cover that would become one of twenty-five annual written chronicles of my mission to live my life while saving it, too. *Well, sweetie,* I began to write that evening, *I've been officially diagnosed with multiple myeloma. I am so sorry because I know it's going to be a tough road for all of us . . .*

Step 2

Meet the Specialists

What Do I Have?

That initial glimpse of a scary diagnosis can be overwhelming. Maybe you're given an ambiguous hypothetical—a preliminary verdict that requires more testing to confirm. Or perhaps your disease is undeniably clear and definitive from the start. Either way, now you have to take a giant step in a new direction, gain your bearings, and then course correct as you surf on this unexpected wave of ups and downs.

Your next step is to meet the specialists—the medical experts who will determine what you have, what stage you're in, and give you an overview about your treatment options. This involves talking to multiple doctors and asking questions about this unwelcome guest who has entered the party of your life. It takes time. Time to reach out to the doctors and get on their schedules. Time to meet with them in person or talk with them via telemedicine. Each will speak their own language from their own training and expertise. Their calendars are tight; on average, oncologists spend about fifteen minutes with each patient. It's frustrating. But know that they are burdened by a busy clinic, onerous bureaucracy, and complicated hospital metrics that frustrate them, too. Be prepared; take someone with you as another set of eyes and ears. And write everything down or use a recording device on a smartphone or tablet.

The Morning after the Diagnosis

"I have something to tell you," I began, as calmly as possible. I'd called my sister, Karen, from the laundry room of our home because I didn't want Paul or Nicole to hear me. My urge to call her was strong and immediate when I learned of my myeloma. After all, she was my identical twin. She'd been my soulmate since birth. We were always together, especially in times of crisis. An unbreakable bond. Once we were able to stand in our individual cribs on wheels, we learned how to jump in a way to push them side by side so we could be as close as possible and rattle on all night to each other. That's how our mother usually found us in the morning.

My fingers nervously played with the coiled cord of the phone as I waited for Karen to pick up. I was composed but shaking, knowing that this news would crush her. She was so far away in Connecticut.

"How are you?" she asked. I could tell she was juggling her young son JJ in her arms as she answered my call. Karen was also pregnant at the time. Unlike me, she'd blink and get pregnant.

"I've had a crazy week. I'm sorry I haven't called."

"That's okay. It's crazy here, too."

"Karen, I don't know how to say this so I'm just going to tell you. I have cancer."

"Oh my God, Kathy. Are you kidding me? What the f—?" She stopped herself from swearing in front of JJ. "What kind?"

I know exactly what she was thinking. She was wondering if this was one of the "better" cancers or if we were going to relive what we just went through with Dad. Was I going to have forever, a few years, or just a few months like him?

"It's called multiple myeloma," I answered. "It's a blood cancer—a cancer of the plasma cells in my immune system. I can't believe it." Our grandmother had had breast cancer and I always assumed that was the cancer I would develop, not something like this. "It's so confusing. Paul and I have been working with the doctors to try and figure it all out."

"Multiple myeloma? I've never heard of it, Kathy."

"Nobody has heard of it. And there's nothing out there to treat it."

"There has to be something," Karen said.

"Honestly, it's bad. Nothing in the pipeline. I checked. It's a cancer that's been neglected for decades." I paused before continuing. "There is this one thing—a stem cell transplant. But it's experimental. And I'm probably too early to even be considered. I'm still trying to figure it all out, but I needed you to know. I have no idea how to tell Mom. I haven't told anyone except you."

"I'm so sorry. But we know how to do this. We've done it before. With Dad."

When my father was diagnosed with renal cell carcinoma, we searched for abstracts; calling doctors and looking for clinical trials proved daunting. There wasn't much. And while I was able to find a trial for him at Sloan Kettering, his cancer had progressed too far for it to make a difference.

"Remember, you're a lot younger than he was, Kathy. You're stronger. I'll start doing some research now." Karen was ready to dive in and help in any way possible. Two sisters with a single mission: not letting one of them die.

Before saying goodbye, she added, "I need to see you right away. I'm going to fly out there as soon as I can." And with just those words, I sensed a bit of relief. Nothing would make me happier than a visit from Karen. She felt so far away. Everyone felt so far away.

After talking with Karen, it was time to call Mom. Like ripping a Band-Aid off, I just said it.

"Mom, I'm really sorry to even have to tell you this after all you've gone through with Dad, but I have cancer."

Mom was a nurse so she got right to it. "What kind?"

"Multiple myeloma." I started explaining this blood cancer when Mom stopped me.

"I know what multiple myeloma is; your grandfather had it."

WTF! How could I not have known that? My grandfather lived with us for years and died in a fire in our home. It was tragic. I had no idea he'd had cancer.

"There was no point in telling you because he was doing okay. And you were young. He lived with it longer than they expected."

My mind immediately went to those endless medical forms I filled out. I never once said I had a grandfather with cancer. Then I thought, if he lived longer than expected, what about me? Maybe I'd inherited a kinder/gentler myeloma? Is this disease even hereditary?

Later that week Karen arrived and we immediately got to work. Like me, Karen had also been premed in college and was comfortable around basic biology and scientific jargon. Now, as a top legal advisor for media giant Time, Inc., research was a great skill of hers. If there was a hospital or doctor who could give me a better chance, she would find them. Her issue would be time. She had a demanding career, a long commute to the city, and a toddler, and she was pregnant. Fitting in cancer research for her sister would not be easy.

Karen went to the local library and pulled anything and everything she could find—from dense scientific papers to a breezy article in *People* magazine. I continued to lean on Searle's medical library, accessing any and every abstract out there on myeloma and drugs being developed to treat it. Sadly, our success rate was not much different from what we found for Dad's kidney cancer. Both were fatal cancers with practically no advancements for treatments. We were feeling the same sense of dread we did two years ago. Every once in a while we would find something new on stem cell transplants or vaccines. We would send those papers back and forth, igniting a glimmer of hope amid the devastating death curves. But in those days of microfiche, fax machines, and plopping nickels into giant copy machines, our work was arduous and frustrating.

My next step was to deal with work, which had been my

everything—perhaps to a fault. It was common to put in a sixty-five-hour week. I loved my job and the people I worked with, and I was laser focused and moving up the ladder. I'd never been late and never missed a meeting. My boss at Searle, Al Heller, was smart, driven, and often intimidating, but also funny and caring. He was the COO at the time and headed for the top position. He once held an off-site summit with his executive team and when the meeting was coming to a close, he asked everyone to write down who they wanted as a mentor. I wrote his name and it was the best move ever. I was shocked that others seemed nervous to do the same. He asked me where I wanted to be in five years; I replied, quite nonchalantly, "In your job."

Okay, that was a bit obnoxious, I grant you, but he took me seriously, saw my potential, and worked with HR to start putting my rotations together. First was worldwide experience and next was running a brand-new sales team in the Midwest region with three hundred people reporting to me. That's the meeting I was leading before the call from Steinmuller. Before cancer. So here I was, on my way, and now everything was coming to a tumultuous halt.

I had called Al's assistant to meet with him and walked up to the quiet executive floor like I'd done so many times. He greeted me wondering why I'd been out. I'd had to call in sick all these days and now I realized he thought I had been interviewing and was resigning.

"Is everything okay?" he asked.

I explained I had been diagnosed with multiple myeloma, once again going through the *it's a blood cancer nobody has heard of . . . based on what I know so far, it is 100 percent fatal . . . and I have about three years to live*. He was in shock, at a loss for words. I didn't sugarcoat anything and knew he appreciated my honesty.

Quickly shifting gears, he said: "We're here for you. Whatever you need."

I was lucky. For now. I knew what I would need most was time. Time to meet with doctors, to get second opinions, to see what new research was happening and how I might become a part of it. I knew from my work at both Merck and Searle that getting to the right hospital, the right doctors, would be my best ticket out.

Al arranged for short-term disability, and we moved my next-in-command up to take my place (temporarily). Most people may not have a boss like Al. And companies might not be as supportive as Searle was. I was grateful to be able to just focus on a game plan.

My first visit after Dr. Slivnik was at Loyola University Medical Center. If there was one thing I knew from working in healthcare, it was the importance of getting a second opinion—even a third. I asked Slivnik for a referral and he suggested I call Dr. Patrick Stiff, Loyola's lead myeloma expert. Slivnik said Loyola was one of the leading centers focused on blood cancers in Chicago. And they were closest, just half an hour from our home. Dr. Stiff was doing research in the space and would be the ideal second opinion. The first call I made, before calling Dr. Stiff's office, was to our insurance company. Again, lucky for me Dr. Stiff was in network and my meeting with him would be covered.

I called Dr. Stiff's office knowing I would need to "sell myself" as a patient. He was clearly a busy man, and I wanted to be seen quickly, to get on his calendar, to learn more. As I went into my name and diagnosis, the receptionist warned me there was a wait and transferred me to the clinical nurse. I paid attention to where she showed interest and built from there. "Hi, my name is Kathy Giusti, I'm thirty-seven and was just diagnosed with multiple myeloma."

"Thirty-seven?" she interrupted. My age seemed to interest her.

"I have a twin," I added.

"Identical? Do you have any other illnesses?"

"None. I'm as healthy as can be—except for this cancer."

"Where do you live?" she continued.

"About half an hour away." Then I added, "My grandfather also had myeloma."

She immediately asked about my insurance, took my information, and scheduled me for the following week.

I was in.

Next was the hassle of getting Stiff the reports from Slivnik—no easy feat back in the days of fax machines and landlines. I literally carried my scans in a huge folder with me. And I had my biopsies in paraffin blocks if anyone wanted those, too.

Dr. Stiff first focused on the fact that my biomarker, my "M-spike," was at a clear Stage I or even Stage II level, which meant treatment. Then he noted my bone marrow biopsy looked like I could be "smoldering," meaning my cancer was slow-growing and didn't necessarily warrant immediate treatment. I'd learned so much already in my personal research about this disease and had read about this possibility in the bookstore, though it was all so ambiguous, convoluted. Stiff also pointed out that Slivnik's X-rays did not show lesions. That was good news, too. Basically, we were all confused. Mixed signals.

Stiff recommended watching and waiting to see if my "M-spike" biomarker stayed stable. Maybe my immune system would keep holding on to fight the cancer. But this whole watch-and-wait idea was foreign to me. Who would think you could have cancer in your body and just leave it there?

On to more second opinions. Karen and I identified several outstanding myeloma experts through our research and I ended up using the same spiel I used with Stiff's office to get appointments with a number of them.

Ken Anderson, a myeloma expert I learned about at Dana-Farber in Boston, spoke with me for nearly an hour. By the end of our call, he was also on the watch-and-wait team.

A transplant center in Seattle said don't wait, on the other hand. They were doing early stem cell transplants in myeloma and believed I would be an excellent candidate. Their conversation with me was convincing as they dared to use the word "cure." But when I called my insurance company, they wouldn't commit to covering a transplant this early and wouldn't give an answer for down the line.

What the fuck.

The advice I was collecting competed for space in my brain. *Take a watch-and-wait approach. Chemo now . . . no, not yet. Undergo a stem cell transplant immediately, then chemo. No, hold off on the transplant. Delaying may be better . . . Sit it out for now . . .* Adding to this maelstrom were astounding requests from some of these myeloma doctors asking me to "take notes" from the other experts and report back as I gathered opinions and ideas for treatment. Like I was a secret courier of intelligence between their separate silos. The disconnects were painfully obvious.

Then some helpful information came along. In her research, Karen ultimately discovered that the Mayo Clinic had the largest database of smoldering patients and was set up to do high-quality diagnostic testing that could better validate where I was on the cancer spectrum. So after weeks of research, calls, and doctors' visits that felt like years, Paul and I headed to Minnesota armed with Karen's and my questions.

Mayo was built with the weather in mind, a campus-like sprawl with underground tunnels and shielded passageways from the icy outdoors as you shuttle from building to building. Getting there was like traveling to the land of Oz through a snowstorm. We flew from Chicago and drove the final ninety minutes past vast farmland, the windshield wipers whisking away snowflakes. It was below zero, the coldest day in a decade. By this point, I'd spent an untold number of hours conducting my research with my sister. Paul helped plan and was at the doctor visits, always driving. Always supportive. It was like trying to complete an endurance race without any training.

Arriving at Mayo, I felt like Dorothy entering the Emerald City. Mayo was this mecca of technology and patient convenience. It's Midwest laid-back, but inside were some of the best systems I'd seen in healthcare. People from all over the world came here. You could tell by their clothes, the many languages they spoke. And all this technology and science was there to serve the patient. To serve me.

When we checked into the clinic, we were handed a personalized schedule for three intense days of scans, biopsies, blood, and urine tests. We would see Dr. Philip Greipp, one of the world's leading experts in multiple myeloma, at the end of day one.

The first day was long and hard, and when we went to see Dr. Greipp I was still a bit groggy from doing the bone marrow biopsy. They had given me an anesthesia, (aptly) dubbed twilight, to put me out. Most centers didn't use twilight because it's expensive and takes longer to go into effect. But it's kinder to the patient and gets a better sample for the doctors. Another plus for Mayo.

Paul and I sat on the wooden benches in the vast hematology waiting room leafing through magazines trying to stay distracted. Paul could feel my frustration rising. Two hours later, we were finally ushered into Dr. Greipp's office. He apologized for the wait, then said he needed to get to the YMCA for his workout. Paul could sense that I was ready to snap this man's head off and shot me the look. Not the best start.

Dr. Greipp explained that his goal was to better understand my staging. While the results of Slivnik's tests looked aggressive, others demonstrated that it might be smoldering, that my immune system was still fighting to keep my cancer in check.

"But how will we know whether I'm smoldering for sure?" I asked, armed with my litany of questions. "What are the extra tests you could do to help us find out? And if I'm smoldering, how long will I stay in that stage? Would I start treatment now?"

From the chair next to me, Paul took my hand and squeezed it in a way that cautioned me to keep it together.

Dr. Greipp waited to make sure I was done. He then explained that, at Mayo, they had additional testing that would better determine the state of my disease—improved scans, a plasma cell labeling index, and even trials looking at other biomarkers that I would be part of. He told me there were no easy answers, but if the tests showed that the myeloma was indeed smoldering, I would have the option to delay treatment with monitoring. Vigilant monitoring.

"Test results first. Then we can talk."

Meeting the Doctors

When your "first" doctor calls to share their suspicions, know that confirming the hypothesis is likely going to take some time. And knowing the stage and specific biology of what you have often means meeting several additional specialists in rapid-fire succession.

I was fortunate that a good internist caught my myeloma early and quickly referred me to the right specialist, a hematologist-oncologist. I was also fortunate that my second opinions were covered by my insurance. Second opinions should be covered, but check first with your insurance company and do not be afraid to push back if you get an initial no. I remember explaining to my insurance company why I needed to go to Mayo. Determining the exact stage of my cancer was essential to making any decisions about my care or my life. I was tenacious and wouldn't take no for an answer. I was also fortunate to have the support of my employer and made sure to keep in constant touch with them. Every day I had off work was a day to conduct research and get the answers we needed.

Flash forward to my more recent cancer experience: When I was diagnosed with breast cancer I was already with a specialist. Knowing I was high risk (more on this later), I was being closely monitored by Dr. Elisa Port, a breast surgeon at Mt. Sinai, a major academic center in New York City. Based on the biopsy, she knew my cancer was very early stage. Once she provided the preliminary results, I was easily moved to appointments with a medical oncologist and radiation oncologist (both at Mt. Sinai as well) to help decide my treatment plan. Each of these doctors has different training, unique knowledge, and fine-tuned expertise. For many women, your diagnosis might start with an OBGYN who sees something on a routine mammogram and refers you to the breast surgeon. Again, many of the appointments and follow-up tests were covered. Still, we did have out-of-pockets that took us by surprise. Look out for this. Make sure you know what you are signing before you sign. And keep asking questions if you're not sure. When you have cancer, the last things you need are unexpected bills. Here are the key WTDs when it's time to meet your second and third opinions.

STEP 2: MEET THE SPECIALISTS

WTDs

Confirm Your Coverage

- X Know your coverage type
- X Know the main details of your plan
- X Pay attention to what you are signing

Prepare for the Specialists

- X Check their bios and hospital affiliations
- X Write your questions in advance
- X Know the difference between specialties

Get Second Opinions

- X Obtain referrals: from your doctor, disease foundation(s), insurance company, and friends
- X Make an appointment: in-person visit or teleconference if possible and appropriate
- X Think about the future role of the second opinion expert: advisor or leader?

WTD 1: Confirm Your Coverage

A survey by the American Cancer Society Cancer Action Network (CAN) has found that nearly one-quarter of respondents had received a surprise bill. Most of these bills were for more than $500—and more than one-fifth of these bills were for $3,000 or more. Those can be crushing costs for many families, especially if they start coming in one after the other. Such a sudden and unexpected financial hit can affect your decisions, whether you choose to see a certain recommended doctor or take a certain treatment. You do not want to have to prioritize cost over care.

✓ *Know your coverage type*

Before making any more appointments, contact your insurance provider to confirm that the centers, doctors, and procedures are covered to treat your condition. Although this can be done through most insurance companies' websites, I encourage you to pick up the phone and speak to a human being. Start with the phone number on the back of your insurance card. If your current healthcare center or doctor is not in network, you'll need to determine where else to go. You absolutely want to minimize any out-of-pocket costs for your care. Here are the three main types of insurance:

→ **Private insurance**: This includes several different subtypes:

   X Individual and family policies with one of the large commercial health insurance companies

   X Group plans through your employer (also usually with one of the large insurance companies)

   X Affordable Care Act (www.healthcare.gov) coverage bought within your state

→ **Within the private insurance realm there are also differences between Health Maintenance Organizations (HMOs) and Preferred Provider Organizations (PPOs)**:

   X HMOs: With an HMO, you choose a primary care doctor who coordinates your healthcare and refers you to specialists within a limited network.

   X PPOs: With a PPO, you have more flexibility in terms of who you can see. You aren't limited to a specific network (though you'll generally have lower out-of-pocket costs if you stay in-network) and you often don't need to go through an internist to see a specialist with a PPO.

X   Many of the large insurance companies offer both HMO and PPO plans. The largest insurance companies today include Kaiser Permanente, Blue Cross Blue Shield, United Health Care, Aetna, and Cigna.

→ **Medicare (www.medicare.gov)**: This is the federal health insurance program for people sixty-five and older and certain younger people with disabilities. It is often used in addition to general health insurance from private companies and comes in four different parts with varying benefits. According to a recent study, "Medicare will account for 70 percent of cancer patients by 2030" and "access to Medicare significantly impacts detection of certain cancers" and "reduces cancer mortality rates."

→ **Medicaid (www.medicaid.gov)**: This is a joint federal- and state-run program designed for people with limited income and resources. People eligible for Medicaid include low-income adults, children, pregnant women, elderly adults, and those with disabilities.

→ **What if you don't have any insurance?** Visit www.HealthCare .gov and click through for information, applications, and state-specific enrollment forms.

✓ *Know the main details of your plan*

To get a sense of your costs going forward, you'll want to be clear about what kinds of insurance you have and what your policies say about out-of-pocket costs:

→ **Copays**: a prespecified contribution toward the cost of doctor visits, medical treatments, drugs, or other covered services

→ **Deductibles**: the prespecified amount you must pay before your insurance kicks in and pays its share of covered services

→ **Out-of-pocket maximums**: the maximum amount, or cap, you will have to pay in a given year before your insurance pays 100 percent of qualified costs

→ **In-network versus out-of-network providers**: In-network providers accept your insurance plan's approved pricing whereas out-of-network providers expect you to pay the difference between their full charge and your plan's preapproved amount. If cost is an issue, you want to find in-network doctors and services wherever possible.

✓ *Pay attention to the forms you sign*

Make sure you're aware of what you are signing when filling out those intake forms at your appointments. You're given the financial parameters and what you could be responsible for should your insurance not afford you coverage. You'll want full disclosure and an understanding of potential out-of-pocket costs. If you have any questions, ask your provider and call your insurance company as well.

WTD 2: Prepare for the Specialists

✓ *Read up on the doctors' bios*

You can do a quick search online to gather background information on the doctors you're seeing. Look up their names, credentials, and specialty. You'll want to know their area of expertise and what it means for you. Also, check to see which hospital they are affiliated with. Is it a hospital near you that you will be comfortable working with?

✓ *Write your questions in advance*

No matter who you're interviewing in the process of determining your diagnosis, the questions are similar:

→ What exactly do I have (e.g., type, subtype, stage)?

→ How many patients have you treated with my specific type of disease?

→ What are my best options for treatment and their risks versus benefits?

→ Which treatment or combination of treatments would you recommend and why?

→ How will these affect my ability to work, travel, perform daily activities/handle responsibilities, etc.?

→ Should I undergo any additional diagnostic tests before we can begin treatment?

→ What kind of timing are we talking about in terms of treatment and recovery?

→ Who else should I see and talk to about my treatment?

✓ *Know the differences between specialties*

Each specialist will bring their own perspective based upon their particular expertise.

→ *Medical oncologists* are like quarterbacks to the cancer game. These doctors will use modern medicine to prescribe anticancer drugs and bring in other types of oncologists and specialists when necessary to add to a comprehensive approach. You may need, for example, a combination of drug therapy, surgery, and radiation. Medical oncologists typically have information about new drugs and clinical trials (see Step 8). They also know how to deliver the infusions. For patients with solid tumors, medical oncologists are the key doctors.

→ *Surgical oncologists* are what their name implies—these doctors perform surgery to remove cancerous cells and abnormal masses. For a long time, these physicians were the primary cancer doctors because there was nothing else to do but attempt to cut out a tumor and nearby tissue in an operation. Surgical oncologists also perform certain types of biopsies to help diagnose and stage cancer, so you know how far the cancer has spread if it has. In some situations, surgical oncologists will perform preventive surgeries.

→ *Hematologist-oncologists* are the cancer doctors who specialize in liquid tumors or cancers found in bodily fluids, such as blood, bone marrow, and lymph. These include blood cancers (e.g., leukemia), cancer of the lymph nodes (e.g., lymphoma), and other parts of the immune system (e.g., multiple myeloma). If your primary care physician suspects you have a liquid cancer, you'll be sent directly to a heme-onc for further testing, diagnosing, and staging.

→ *Radiation oncologists* (rad-oncs) are the experts at radiation therapy, which is the use of high-energy X-rays or other particles to destroy cancer cells. Depending on your cancer, you may need additional testing to decide whether you need radiation or not. For my breast cancer, a radiation oncologist checked my tissue to see how responsive it would be to radiation. Turns out I wasn't a good candidate for effective radiation, and that fact alone helped me in my decision-making process.

WTD 3: Get Second Opinions

✓ ***Obtain referrals from your doctor, disease foundation(s), insurance company, and friends***

Every specialist you consult with, ask for more referrals or other people to consult with, any additional testing to consider, and their perspective on overall sense of timing. Don't be shy! This is your life—no matter how awkward you may feel. You won't alienate a doctor by looking elsewhere. Doctors give second opinions all the time. It's routine. Second and third opinions are essential to your survival (and your quality of life along the way). Extra opinions are especially helpful if the first one didn't sit well with you. Truly, you can never have too much information, and the input you gather from all these specialists will ultimately help you further frame and fine-tune your decisions and overall plan. Here are some tips:

→ Start by asking each doctor you meet with to recommend who else in the area works in this space. The referral can be within your doctor's camp (affiliated hospital or center) or elsewhere.

→ Return to your online research and check the foundations that focus on your specific disease. Many of these foundations provide doctor recommendations and referrals.

→ Check other accredited sites that feature doctor finders as well. For example, the directory of Castle Connolly's "Top Doctors" (www.castleconnolly.com) finds the best-in-class across all major specialties and most major cities in the country.

→ Ask a trusted friend. Never underestimate the power of word of mouth. Do you have friends that have your condition? Do they have doctors they liked? Ask people to make introductions (better than cold calling). But remember, just because one patient had a great experience at one center for their specific cancer does not mean it's going to be ideal for what you have or what you need.

✓ **Make an appointment: in-person visit or teleconference if possible and appropriate**

Let your personal resources guide you in choosing where to go for extra opinions, especially if there are geographic limitations and you cannot travel hundreds or thousands of miles away. You should be able to find at least one or two extra opinions within your local area, and others may offer telemedicine.

✓ ***Think about the future role of the second opinion expert: advisor or leader?***

Once you've gotten your second or third opinion, you then decide who will take the lead and who will be your backup advisor and reinforcement. You may, for instance, want the doctor who has great acumen for your cancer (but a less-than-ideal bedside manner) to take your lead with the local oncologist who is delivering your daily care and much more accessible.

Reminder: you're not choosing your final doctors yet (we'll talk about that in Part 2). The doctors that diagnose you may not be the doctors who treat you long term. Think of this as an interview process. Whom do you like working with? Do you like the office? What's the gestalt? Are the nurses and nurse practitioners kind and helpful? Where are you most comfortable (community hospital or designated "Center of Excellence")? Is the facility built around your needs as a patient? While talking to these doctors, you may begin to see who you want as your lead—someone who will stay with you through your journey.

IN CONVERSATION WITH MICHAEL SHERMAN

former Chief Medical Officer at Point32Health

A Yale-trained physician with an MBA from Harvard, Dr. Sherman is a well-respected expert in the insurance realm. He has worked in every part of the healthcare ecosystem, with an intense focus on the payor side. Most people think (and worry) about their coverage upon a diagnosis, so I was eager to speak to him about matters of insurance.

Q. What do cancer patients need to know about health insurance upon a cancer diagnosis?
A.   Your first order of business is to find out *who* is your primary health insurance. Most cancer patients are over the age of

sixty-five and will be covered by Medicare, and approximately half of those beneficiaries are enrolled in Medicare Advantage Plans. In fact, Medicare beneficiaries account for more than half of all new cancer cases and that number will continue to rise. The rest rely on private, commercial insurance, with a small percentage (about 15 percent) enrolled in Medicaid. Whatever primary insurance you have, it's critical that you pay attention to your coverage as you do your research and find doctors who are covered by your payor. Even patients enrolled in Medicare Advantage Plans need to ask questions about who is in network with their insurer. Your payor—member services—should be your first call. The number is usually right on the back of your insurance card or you can find it online. You'll want to be in constant contact with them and know how to get preauthorized for anything as you move through diagnostics and into treatment. Note that for people who are transitioning into Medicare upon turning sixty-five, which can happen in the middle of a cancer journey, make sure you start your research six months in advance to find the right blend of coverage that may include supplemental plans.

Q. What is the best way to work with your insurance company? What are the pitfalls to be aware of?

A. Financial toxicity or unexpected bills are often a result of not reading the fine print and asking questions. Insurance companies are investing more money into the service side—having people that can answer the tough questions in easy-to-understand nuggets. People tend to focus on monthly premiums only and not all the moving parts to their coverage—until they are sick. First, you want to know what kind of plan you have—are you in an HMO or PPO? What does that mean? For example, do you need to go through your primary care to see your specialist, which is common when you're in an HMO? Do you need prior authorization? Are there geographic limits? Are all the doctors you're seeing (or will be seeing) in your network? What are the copays/coinsurance, deductibles, and out-of-pocket maximums? And if something is not covered, have your healthcare provider call for you. This is why it's important to have a doctor who will push for you and who is knowledgeable about your insurance—about what payors do and don't do.

Q. What if someone gets hit with an unexpected bill? What should they do?

A. If something goes wrong with billing, don't be afraid to speak up and escalate. The problem may not have been on your end. Call the insurance company first and then work with the hospital billing office. If you need to, file a formal complaint (what's called a "grievance") using the online form provided by the insurance company. It's important to keep asking if there is a case manager who can support you and your specific needs. And there will be times when they need to hear directly from your physician. Make sure you have an office that will go to bat for you.

❋

"It's Smoldering."

On that third day at the Mayo, when it was finally time for our exit interview and the results, Paul and I sat in Dr. Greipp's office while he was finishing a call. The walls, with their framed accolades and photos, spoke of his athletic accomplishments in addition to his medical distinctions. Dr. Greipp had been a decorated rower in his youth and had finished the Twin Cities Marathon with both of his sons a few years previously. As I sat there with my eyes wandering, I was trying to prepare myself for the worst. Cutting off my train of thought, he hung up the phone, smiled at me, and said, "We have almost every test back, Kathy. Your scans are clean, your kidneys are strong, and your labeling index is low. That's pretty good news. Still, your bone marrow came in with fifteen percent plasma cells and your M-spike remains high." (These once-foreign terms were now part of my everyday vocabulary.) "Based on our data, you will clearly get active myeloma, but you are not quite there yet. That gives you options. We could start talking treatment options now, or you could wait on treatment." He paused before adding, "As long as you stay closely monitored."

Once again, the choice would be mine. There were plenty of patients in my situation that would move. I decided not to. Paul and I had a big decision yet to make.

Step 3

Rethink What Matters

What Do I Need?
What Do I Want?

Most people who face cancer remember the exact day and time their diagnosis was confirmed. Their life is instantly divided in two: life "Before Cancer" and life "After Cancer." They pine for the days Before Cancer when they took their health for granted, when they weren't consumed by doctor's appointments, needle sticks, and paperwork.

It's okay to mourn what you've lost. It's important to do so. But it's also important to acknowledge where you are, to accept that life has changed, and to begin thinking about where you want to be now, in six months, in a year or two. In this step, it's time to take stock of what you need and what you want. And to fully understand how those needs and wants impact those you love.

It starts with your needs. They probably feel immediate to you now. What do you need just to get through the testing and the treatments? Time? Money? Family? Insurance? Employment? Who will drive you to appointments? How will you pay your deductible? Who will cover your shift at work? Who will watch your children or help your parents? Who will help maintain the household?

But more importantly, think about your wants. Don't miss the opportunity you have now, right now, to sit quietly, by yourself, and write out what you want. Most people would not say that their diagnosis was "the best thing that ever happened to them." But for many, a health crisis has a hidden benefit—it forces you to go deep within yourself to begin accepting your new reality and its implications on those you love. If you can "sit in it," what's important comes into clearer focus. What would a good day look like? Who are you spending it with? Is there something you still want to see? Something you still want to say or do?

I would venture to guess the majority of people don't take themselves through a personal "reset" unless they are facing their own mortality. Why? The busyness of life for one. But here's the bigger reason: It takes tremendous discipline and personal honesty. You may have to accept that you didn't yet accomplish what you wanted in your career. You may realize you worked too hard and don't have strong relationships to lean on. You're not alone. But now it's time to ask yourself tough, sometimes insufferable questions about what matters most moving forward. Then you have to recognize who else your reset impacts and bring them into the conversation. This is an important step that cannot be skipped.

Back to Work

I was back working at Searle. Turns out when Mayo confirmed my cancer as smoldering (even if it was "high-risk" smoldering), it meant they deemed me physically capable of working and my short-term disability ended. To our insurance company, *watch and wait* meant *watch and work.* And while Al Heller had been a thoughtful, tireless advocate as I completed my diagnostic research, he had a company to run and I'd been a productive direct report. I'm also sure he thought work would be a good distraction for me. Bottom line, our insurance was through me and working in healthcare, it was a good plan. We needed insurance; I needed to return to work.

But my time with Nicole and endless conversations about my seemingly inevitable death had changed me. I had come to realize how much I loved being home with Nicole without the distractions of a high-level, high-stress, fast-paced job hanging over me. From the moment she was born, Nicole brought such joy to our lives—always smiling, reaching for our fingers or a strand of hair, even quickly learning to sleep through the night. At eighteen months, she was all play with her favorite stuffed animals, puzzles, simple art projects, or strolls through the neighborhood. She gave us so much happiness that Paul and I quickly realized we'd waited way too long to start our family. Having put myself through school, racking up significant debt along the way, I felt compelled to get ahead. But now, it was time to face reality. Despite an incredible ride, despite having finally paid off my loans, despite being on one of the final rotations toward one of the top roles in one of the best companies in the country, I was staring at "three years to live." My career was done. I would never be the first woman anything. I had a job. And that job served one purpose: It provided necessary health insurance for me and our family. And it was here, right here, that I should have written my wants down on paper and looked at them every single day. My first and only wants were to keep our family safe and happy, and to create beautiful memories that would live on long after I was gone.

Thoughts about having another child still stalked me. We had always planned to have three children. And the time we were spending together as a family only confirmed my heart was still where Paul and I had left off Before Cancer. Now I wanted to give Nicole what I always had in Karen—a sibling, a friend, a soulmate in life. Cancer did not interrupt my dream—it only amplified it. It was an ache I could not ignore or pretend wasn't there. I was keenly aware of my imminent death, but I needed to live like I was going to live.

One night soon after returning home from Mayo, I caught sight of Paul in Nicole's nursery from the hallway. He was sitting in the rocking chair (bought for me), holding sleepy Nicole in his lap as they gently rocked back and forth. He'd just finished reading *The Very Hungry Caterpillar* to her as she dozed off. I stopped at the door to listen . . . and to think. It had been a long day that was now ending in a bittersweet moment that cemented my resolve. When I slipped into the room, I broke Paul's gaze from where it had been directed out the window, at nothing.

"I'm sorry," I whispered.

"Why? Sorry for what?" He looked up at me with his warm, brown eyes.

"I can't help but think I did this to myself. Always working. Stressing my system."

"Kathy, you didn't *do* anything." He was desperate for me to believe him. Without jostling Nicole, he reached for my hand across the arm of the rocking chair. "Your grandfather had this disease. Your father died of cancer. You just got dealt a bad genetic hand. That's all. You play the hand you're dealt." He flashed me a secure smile as tears rolled down my face. "You can't talk like this, honey. There's no reason to play the blame game."

Nicole shifted in his arms. He dropped his voice, still looking at me as if I had to believe him. "Kathy, we will get through this. We need to have hope."

I nodded and smiled. I wanted him to see that I heard him, that I believed him.

"I still want to have another child, Paul—for you, and for her. You both deserve that, even if it's the last thing I do," I said.

"We'll see."

"It hurts too much to see you two alone. I can't leave you alone. I can't. If we have a chance, let's take it."

"What if that path makes your cancer worse?"

"That's a risk I would gladly take," I said.

In my journal later that night I sat quietly with my feelings and wrote honestly:

> I look at you both and say I must stay strong. While I'm
> scared of the many paths this journey can take us, I need to

stay focused on the one that is best for our family. I can see
Daddy braiding your hair, taking you to school, and coaching
your teams. I see you doing it all with a wonderful sidekick
like I always had with Karen. You deserve a sibling, a best
friend, a partner in crime.

For me, the journal was a blank sheet of paper. A private place
where I could gather and clarify my innermost thoughts. I was writing to Nicole, but when I look back, I see in many ways I was also
writing to myself.

Writing on a blank sheet of paper in the face of a problem would
become a vital ritual throughout my journey, both to document
what I needed to take care of and to shape how my priorities would
be aligned. Little did I realize then how much my journal entries
would come back to me, an unexpected gift from the not-so-distant
past. The writing took on a life of its own. Nothing had a more powerful influence over my thinking and my understanding about what
I wanted—what my loved ones needed—in the wake of the diagnosis
than my journaling. My entries articulated my deepest wants, informed my toughest decisions, and inspired me to move forward. I
could rest once I'd done everything humanly possible to leave them
in a good, safe, and happy place. Once we'd created memories they
could hold on to. The want was much more than about me—it was
about knowing the people I loved would be okay when I was gone.
My mind could be at peace amid the unfairness of my circumstances.
I did not want to be a burden on anyone, but watching Paul read to
Nicole that night as I lived with an ambiguous death sentence placed
me in a crucible of sorts—one that repeatedly compelled me to take
risks and to keep asking what I wanted personally and emotionally.
What. Do. You. Want?
My dreams needed to be reimagined. And the clock was ticking.
As I sat in my fear, sorrow, and frustration, I continued to journal.
It was my sanctuary as well as my outlet. It was a compulsion that

became my compass. And because I was writing, I was feeling what I was thinking—naming it and beginning to face it.

Early the next morning, while everyone was still sleeping, I pulled the Yellow Pages out from the kitchen drawer where it sat by the phone. That four-inch-thick book of phone numbers would be the one place to tell me if a fertility clinic was even nearby. I wasn't sure what type of physician to look up. And then I saw a small, boxed ad under the hospital section for the Highland Park Hospital Fertility Clinic. It was an omen. Actually, a miracle. The hospital was on my ride to Searle. Maybe I could juggle work, cancer, *and* IVF.

Before dialing the clinic, I had two other calls to make. First, Dr. Greipp. I caught him early before his day started.

"Remember how they found my cancer? During a potential fertility workup?"

It was obvious where I was going. But before he could get his words in, I sped ahead and broached the subject. "Okay, don't say I'm crazy. I know the enormity of this disease, but I have to ask: How might pregnancy impact it?"

He listened quietly, waiting a beat before responding. "Maybe it would be best to see how 'stable' your disease is first? To wait six months and watch the test results?"

"But six months is a long time to wait." All I could think was that my three years had already ticked away to two and a half.

He then explained there was no data on pregnancy and smoldering myeloma, that nobody could be sure what would happen. "What if the pregnancy accelerates the disease? Anything's possible."

"I accept that," I told him. Losing a few months would be worth it if I could leave a healthy child for Paul, a healthy sibling for Nicole.

"Is Paul on board with this decision?" It was the right question to ask. There was no way I could do this alone.

"Yes," I said, knowing Paul had his concerns.

There was another calculated pause before he said, "Kathy, your tests look pretty good. You're a smoldering myeloma patient, and your immune system is behaving for now. You might actually have more time to play with than other patients."

"If ever there were a couple to take this risk, it is us," I assured him.

"I know enough about you to know if you're adamant, you're going to do this," he said, his tone softening a bit in slow surrender. "Just keep me posted on all your appointments. I want to help." Now I knew why Dr. Greipp kept folks like me waiting for their appointments. It wasn't that he needed to be at the gym, it was that he wanted to be there when his patients needed him, not just for their needs, but for their wants.

The next call was to my mom. I needed to say my plan out loud to someone other than Paul or a doctor. Declaring my wishes only made them more real, more attainable, and more immediate. My mother was a woman of brutal honesty. I knew she'd tell me exactly what she thought regardless of how it would make me feel. After a minute of small talk, I got to the point.

"I want to run something by you," I started. "I know this may sound crazy but, even with the cancer, my wish to have another child hasn't gone away."

"Well, of course it hasn't," she returned matter-of-factly. "That's not crazy at all."

Not crazy—the words echoed in my head. You just assume people will think you're being irrational, or irresponsible, or selfish. But then you say it out loud, and they understand.

"This isn't all about me, Mom. It's about Nicole and Paul."

"Honey, you're good at making these decisions. You and Paul can do this."

That's all I needed to hear. My mom's positivity and practicality infused me with even more confidence to move forward. She wasn't someone to feign optimism or pretend to support me if she truly thought I was acting foolish and reckless. Now it was time to act. Now I was ready to call the clinic.

After one short ring, a receptionist answered and, hearing the complexity of my case, she quickly got me on with the nurse who helped run the program.

"Yes, it's absolutely worth talking with Dr. Marut," the nurse replied. (Another person who didn't think I was crazy.) "We won't know, of course, until we have all the information, but we deal with cancer patients often. Let me see how fast we can get you in."

Dr. Edward Marut was the reproductive endocrinologist who ran the fertility clinic. Within the week I was sitting in his office as he reviewed my health record.

"The issue is both your age [*Ugh, why had I waited so long to do this?*] and the impact of your disease," he said bluntly. "While you may be in watch-and-wait mode, we have no idea how pregnancy will impact your disease or how your disease will impact your ability to get pregnant."

"So we don't know my chances?" I asked. I was eyeing the poster above his desk comparing age to likelihood of success.

"Nobody knows in this situation. We can't give you the odds of this working out, but there are a few things we can try."

"What do we need to do?"

"First, we run some tests."

More tests. And like that, I was thrown into yet another club I hadn't known existed. The world of infertility is one of fear and loneliness. It seems everyone you know just looks at their partner and gets pregnant. Paul and I were thirty-six years old when we had Nicole. We didn't need IVF at the time, but my career focus had pushed us into a corner and the clock was already ticking. Cancer only made the clock tick faster.

Every morning I would show up at the clinic at seven a.m. trying to be first in line to get tested before I started a full day at work. I'd sit on the floor outside Marut's office with my Dunkin' Donuts coffee. It was dark, chilly, and quiet. My fellow club mates would show up as well. While none of us wanted to chat, sometimes we did. Where are you in the process? How many tries have you done? How many embryos did you get? How much money have you spent? Everyone had her story, like the woman who'd sold her car for a final shot at a child, or the woman who'd just been declared in remission for her lung cancer and was now going for a second child. As I went through the injections and endless ultrasounds, I was constantly reminded I could go through all of this, and it *still* might not work.

With little time to waste, I went rapidly from routine injections to boosting my egg production to the much more challenging process of in vitro fertilization. I was blown away by the science. Doctors used a new technique known as intracytoplasmic sperm injection (ICSI), which had been invented just five years before. Now, a single sperm could fertilize the egg in a petri dish to create embryos. The embryos could then be graded in terms of viability to help decide which were optimal for implantation. All I could think was, I'm dying and yet we are creating life in this extraordinary way. Still, there was a 70 percent chance it wouldn't work. And the process was intense. Paul was giving the injections; I was traveling for work. The hormones were strong, my emotions stronger. When the first round didn't work, I was devastated. With no time to waste, we tried again. Implantation followed by miscarriage, followed by implantation, followed by nothing. It was distressing. Fertility treatments were taking a toll on me and taking me away from Nicole. Paul was increasingly worried about what pumping myself with hormones would do to the cancer. We decided we'd had enough. I wanted to spend what good years I had left with Paul and Nicole, not doing more tests and treatments. We agreed to try one last time, but that would be it. Hard stop if it didn't work. Accept that it's not meant to be.

On the way to the clinic for the final embryo transfer, we stopped at St. Patrick's, the church we'd been attending for years. It was a beautiful church supported by our kind, gentle priest, Father McNulty. Paul was raised a Catholic, attending church every Sunday, and St. Patrick's was the one place where he felt comfortable on this journey, where we both felt comfortable. The door was open. We quietly went in, lit a candle, and prayed.

What Do You Need, What Do You Want?

After being diagnosed with myeloma, we had immediate needs, from insurance to childcare to work. The needs were obvious to Paul and me. The wants, less so. I only started to think about my wants with that moment in the bookstore when I saw that journal with the yellow-orange sunflower by the register. Right then, it hit me that I wanted to write to Paul and Nicole. I wanted to share every detail of our short three years. I wanted to express how much I loved them and would miss them. But sitting and writing in those first pages of that first journal late at night or in the early morning brought so much more. Yes, I mourned the loss of my career. And yes, I accepted that those tuition bills and sixty-five-hour weeks were now sunk costs and lost time. But I loved each day with Paul and Nicole and cherished every new game we played or outing we took. Now I had only two wants: to keep our family safe and happy, and to build memories that would last.

By the time I was diagnosed with breast cancer, everything had changed. I was very aware of the toll my long cancer journey had taken on Paul. I wasn't sure I could ask any more from him. I wanted off the cancer roller coaster as quickly as possible. I was now writing in my twenty-fifth journal and yet my North Star was exactly the same. Keep our family safe and happy. Build memories that will last forever. I just wish I had kept that North Star where I would have seen it every day in between. Keep your North Star front and center on your journey. Come back to it every day. It's the one gift a cancer diagnosis may give you.

Your personal reset will no doubt look nothing like mine, but here are some key WTDs to guide you.

STEP 3: RETHINK WHAT MATTERS
WTDs

List Your Needs and Wants
 X What you need to give up (and mourn)
 X What you need to ease the journey
 X What you want on the other side

Say It Out Loud
 X Share your wishes with someone you trust
 X Broaden your circle of those who can help
 X Consider outside support

Establish Your North Star!
 X Decide what's most important
 X Commit, sign, and post

WTD 1: List Your Needs and Wants

Using whatever form of writing or recording tool you prefer (blank sheet of paper, journal, notepad, laptop, or app on your phone), start answering some important questions in a comfortable place where you can be alone with your thoughts. If getting into this zone means walking, driving, or doing some activity on autopilot that's calming, that's fine. Self-awareness is essential here to go deep and extract your gems—both gems of your lightness and the dark places. And free associate! You can correct and edit your thoughts later. Here are some prompts:

✓ *What you need to give up (and mourn accordingly)*
   You are coming to grips with the reality that your new "post-diagnosis" life means change. They may be small, temporary changes like cutting back on exercise or having to miss business or

social events. Or they may be more significant, such as a change in career plans or family dynamic. Whatever changes you're facing, it is important to accept that these losses have happened and to recognize the impact they will have on your life. It's okay, even critical, to mourn these losses. Acknowledging them, naming them, putting them down on paper, will help you move on from what you have to give up. And be patient with yourself. Moving beyond grief takes time, and there is no set timeline for how long it should—or will—take.

✓ *What you need to ease the journey*

Now that you've listed what you need to give up, move to what you need going forward. This will clear your mind for thinking out ahead to what you want. What comes to mind when you force yourself to be quiet with your eyes closed? What's keeping you up at night? What worries you the most? Is it your family? Your job? Your medical coverage? Your transportation? Your side effects? Your physical appearance? These are all completely normal. Put them down on paper. Again, free associate.

✓ *What you want on the other side*

Next, move to your wants. What are your hopes and dreams now? Is there something you want to accomplish, or a way you want to be remembered? Is there a place or an event you want to see? Who do you want to spend time with? Do you have regrets that you might be able to address now or in the near future? This is a good, honest time to take honest note of the things that live in the depths of your mind.

This exercise can be intimidating, and that's okay. Just as you sit in the reality of your diagnosis, you now sit in all the thoughts that explode to the surface. No sooner did I learn I had a rare blood cancer with no cure than I began to beat myself up for waiting so long to have children and for working so damn hard. I had to face my potential legacy and go so far as to question if I even had one yet. So, ask yourself: What might you lose and what might you be able to do or keep? What regrets can you reverse? What can you gain control of now in preparation for your "new" future?

WTD 2: Say It Out Loud

Once you have framed your needs and wants internally, talk them out honestly with others. By speaking your thoughts out loud, they become real. Certain ones will rise to the top, others you may realize are not as important to you, or necessary. And talking them through will help you build clarity about what matters and what's possible.

✓ *Share your wishes with someone you trust*
Start with someone you trust, ideally someone who does not have skin in the game or an agenda of their own. They can help you organize, prioritize, balance pros and cons, and articulate your thoughts and ideas better and know the implications on others. I initially spoke with my mother about having another child. She didn't say I was crazy. She gave me the confidence to keep going. And to keep asking questions and searching for optimism. If you find the right person, they can help you to build and keep building on your war chest of wishes and the confidence to go after them.

✓ *Broaden your circle of those who can help*
After your first conversation with someone you trust, seek out others you might feel comfortable talking to. It could be a friend, a coworker, a social worker, a patient peer. If you know someone who's been through a similar experience, they might have thoughts or ideas that would shed new light on your plans. If you

have a boss you know you can trust, who will be receptive to a conversation about your diagnosis, have that dialogue.

✓ *Consider outside support*

Not everyone is comfortable talking about their diagnosis and life plans with friends and colleagues. If you run into a roadblock, there is always outside help. Your hospital will have social workers, nonprofits like CancerCare and the American Cancer Society can help you find support, and your disease-focused nonprofit might have navigators or mentors to provide thoughts. And if you're part of a church or local community organization, reach out to them. They will often have designated people to counsel members.

WTD 3: Establish Your North Star!

✓ *Decide what's most important*

It's time to take your list of needs and prioritize them. Do the same for your wants. Your caregiving team can support you on those prioritized needs. But really think through your priority wants. Narrow it down to one or two. That is your North Star. Go for it knowing that it might involve others and you will need to bring them into the fold.

✓ *Commit, sign, and post*

Once you have your North Star, put it where you'll see it every day. It could be on a kitchen refrigerator, the bathroom mirror, or your desktop computer. Put it where you can't forget it and where you can't ignore it. Every time you make a decision going forward, whether about your care or your life, make sure you ask yourself "Does this decision help me get to my North Star?" And if it does, move ahead. But if it doesn't, you need to ask yourself whether you should change the decision or change your North Star.

HIGHLIGHTS FROM MAYA SHANKAR'S INTERVIEW WITH ADAM GRANT

psychologist and author of the bestselling
Think Again

Dr. Maya Shankar's popular podcast *A Slight Change of Plans* often features experts to talk about the science of human behavior and how we can live more fulfilling lives. Shankar, a PhD in cognitive neuroscience, served as the first behavioral science advisor to the United Nations and was a senior advisor in the Obama White House. I love listening to the inspiring stories and wisdom shared on her podcast that illustrate the power of change—especially when that change is forced upon you. One conversation in particular that stood out to me was between Maya and Adam Grant, a popular professor at Wharton who teaches how to "rethink assumptions" and find greater meaning in life. Here are some insights from their exchange that will help you rethink what matters now.

Be willing to rethink

Resetting your wants and needs in life is hard because it likely entails a shift in beliefs. This can result in a struggle, and according to Grant, your intelligence can get in the way—the smarter you are, the more challenging it can be to revise your values, or what you think is important. To combat this challenge, it may help to avoid overintellectualizing your reset. Be open-minded about your value system and "be willing to change those fundamental beliefs." Values are not "set in stone." They are fluid and move with the information and facts you have at the time.

Leverage the power of doubt in yourself

There are a lot of unknowns when it comes to a cancer diagnosis. You might doubt yourself—and your future—more than ever before. And that doubt may intrude and cloud your thinking as you rethink what matters. On a positive note, there are surprising benefits to having doubts and feeling ill-confident. According to Grant, who references Professor Basima Tewfik's work studying how often people doubt themselves, when your confidence is lower than your competence, you're more likely "to work smarter, to learn new things . . . and be more receptive to listening to other people." That last point is key. As you wrestle with doubt and map out your needs and wants, keep your ears open and take in what others have to say. There will be blanks to fill that might come from other people.

Detach your current self from your old self

The line between Before Cancer and after your diagnosis can feel so strong that it fuels an identity crisis. You can't ever go back to Before Cancer, and now you have to reset your life going forward. But here's something interesting, according to Grant: Studies show that people who feel "derailed" can end up feeling happier after a period of being unsettled. Sounds counterintuitive, but the thinking is that the unsettling period leads people to a place where they can let go of old ideas about who they wanted to be. Those old ideas won't hold you back. As you articulate your new needs and wants and establish your North Star, think from where you are in this moment—not Before Cancer.

"You're Pregnant!"

On September 7, eight months after my diagnosis and several cycles of trying to get pregnant, I was waiting for the phone to ring. I had stopped by Dr. Marut's office that morning for a blood test to see if I was pregnant. Knowing this was our final attempt, my anxiety had firmly set in. It was around eight p.m. when Paul called me. I had put Nicole to bed early and was sitting on our bed catching up on some reading for work when the phone rang. Paul had been working late.

"I have amazing news for you," he announced. "Dr. Marut just called me. You're pregnant."

I jumped off the bed and screamed into the phone, right into his ear.

To this day, I don't know why Paul got that call rather than me. Still, I felt like the luckiest woman alive. After all the hurdles, we were ecstatic. (But I was also wary knowing a miscarriage could happen again.) The next morning, Paul was out the door early. He left a note for me on the kitchen counter: *It wasn't a dream. Love you!*

Paul and I lived quietly in this space of good news, just the two of us. The only person I told was Karen. The only person Paul told was Father McNulty. In the back of our minds, we believed our prayers had made the difference. With no family in Chicago, St. Patrick's was our community. Paul was a lector there, and I worked in the nursery while watching Nicole. I had converted to Catholicism with Father McNulty just one year before my diagnosis. We were not just parishioners; we were friends.

Father McNulty understood the challenges we were facing. He also understood how those challenges just got a whole lot more challenging. He recommended we talk with his friend Jack Clark. Jack had helped other parish families move through transitions like ours. Clearly, having another child was the first of many new steps we now needed a plan for. Time for another blank sheet of paper.

Step 4

Make Your Action Plan

How Do We Get It Done?

Now that your needs and wants are clear and stated, the fourth step in any survival kit is to build a plan to get it done. Be sure to keep it simple. Start with your top priority needs and wants and determine what and who it will take to get you there, and in what time frame. Then you can adjust for variables, uncertainties, and unanswerable questions. How will your day-to-day needs be answered? Your family's? How will you manage your job?

This does not need to be a detailed multipage business plan. It can be a one-page punch list. What are your core must-dos to reach your North Star? What changes do you have to make to your current life and what can you keep the same? Who will you need for support along the way, and how will you support them back? What must you do now, and what might wait for a more convenient moment? And how will you adapt if and when the plan needs to change along the way?

Your plan can be supplemented by a calendar and call list. It can be managed by someone other than you. The better you plan and the wider you cast your net, the less pressure placed on one or two people. And if you only have one person, that's okay, you can get outside support as well. Remember, once you make your plan, it's best to give everyone time and clear direction on how to help.

A Blank Sheet of Paper

On the way to see Jack Clark, the counselor that Father McNulty had recommended, I stopped off at the Starbucks across the street from Jack's office and spent the thirty minutes before our meeting sitting with the single question he had asked Paul and me to come in ready to answer: Where do we see ourselves in six months, one year, maybe two? Clearly, he had grasped the severity of myeloma.

With just a pen from my purse and a brown paper napkin from the canister, I started writing. I loved this kind of exercise; it was right up my alley to organize my thoughts on a blank sheet of paper, even on a flimsy napkin. The challenge was being realistic. It took five or six napkins to get there, but my scribble ended up being a simple list: Deliver a healthy baby; surround our family with love and support; build memories that would last.

Jack got a clear picture of Paul and me from this first discussion. With my constant journaling, all I did was think about the future. I was able to give him my three priorities on a single paper napkin. But for each priority, I already had a long mental list of WTDs to reach those goals. It would take dozens of napkins to contain what was in my head. Paul, on the other hand, didn't put anything on paper. Not because he didn't care, but because he cared so much. His wife was carrying his child and likely going to die. He wanted to live for today and looking ahead was too much. When Jack asked him about my list, Paul simply nodded. He would put my needs over his.

Jack quickly zeroed in on my priorities: what was needed, the timing, and who could help. We slowly went through each.

Delivering a healthy baby meant balancing my high-risk pregnancy with high-risk myeloma. It meant working through the medical issues with Dr. Greipp and Dr. Marut and doing everything possible to take care of myself. It meant double, if not triple the number of appointments and lab tests while I was still busy at work. We had amazing childcare for Nicole and neighborhood friends who could help but they were employed full-time. We had no family nearby—none. Everyone was a flight away.

That brought us to my second priority—surrounding our family with love and support. No sooner did I share the urge to go back home to Connecticut than Paul concurred that it'd be ideal to live closer to his parents as well. He adored his mother and father and missed them tremendously while we lived in Chicago. Each of the most important people in our lives—my sister and his parents, respectively—happened to live ten minutes apart. No matter what happened to me, Paul was happy to be near the people who could be helpful and supportive. Once we started thinking this way, we became excited about discussing towns and homes we could afford. But the next task became planning for how we could achieve this life-changing goal. I would be leaving my job and Paul would be the breadwinner, the insurance keeper. Paul had left his big company job to start his own company. It was his passion job. Would he have to leave it behind and go to work for a big company again? What was realistic given our circumstances? And how could we best prepare for evolving circumstances?

"What makes you the most nervous?" Jack asked, careful to look at each of us squarely in the eyes. "What is the greatest challenge— the biggest hurdle to moving to Connecticut?"

"Selling our home," I chimed in. "Leaving my job. Saying goodbye to my career and peers for good." I paused, then blurted out: "And running out of time to get this all done."

"Making sure we are okay financially and that Kathy has the best doctors," Paul added. He never talked about what he would be giving up. My cancer would always come first.

"Well, that's a start," Jack said assuredly. "Let's make the most of our time and go from here. We'll make a list of all the things you think you must do to execute this plan . . ."

Our situation was unique and fortunate. And I get it. I was lucky to have a husband who was willing to do anything and everything to support our growing family. Not everyone has a built-in support network, or even an opportunity to consider such drastic changes in location and lifestyle. Then there's the money, insurance, and access to healthcare that we had. These aspects, too, were easier for us to navigate than they are for others. Everyone's circumstances are different, therefore their options—and the choices they must make because of them—will be different. Uprooting yourself from where you live based on a diagnosis is not typically feasible or practical. Nor is it even the right option for most people. But for us, it was the path that made the most sense. We didn't have any family nearby in the Chicago area. My journals reveal how much I imagined I'd have to rely on my sister, someone who could help me follow through on my plan and dive into the deep end with me. And when I died, at least Karen could help fill the role of surrogate mother. She'd be right there. Paul would also need his own backup support through his parents. Because I might not live much longer than three years, I felt compelled to set everything up for that possible fate. I followed the old adage of "prepare for the worst and hope for the best." I assumed my life would be short and made plans accordingly.

But I also wanted to live. At this point in my journey, I knew that my sister was an option for a possible stem cell transplant, so it made sense to be near her for that inevitability. I also knew that Connecticut would bring me closer to exceptional myeloma care. I had initially connected with Ken Anderson while seeking out a second opinion and appreciated his knowledge and calm approach. I had met him again at a leading myeloma meeting he was chairing for the International Myeloma Workshop (IMW) in Boston and was impressed with his ability to bring the small myeloma community together. Stationed at Dana-Farber Cancer Institute in Boston, he would now be a reasonable drive from Connecticut.

Paul and I had met as students at Harvard Business School (HBS). I had applied on a whim never believing I'd be accepted. I spent my first year terrified, feeling like I had a case of imposter syndrome. I'd never read a case study; my only business class had been a nighttime accounting course I took while working my first job out of college at Merck. Paul, on the other hand, was confident and prepared. I studied excessively and kept more to myself; he studied just enough, socialized, and knew everyone on campus.

But I was very newly single—only a few weeks out from leaving a relationship that had just crossed the five-year mark. I wasn't even thinking of jumping back into dating, but the conversation kept going with every classmate saying the same thing: "KD, he is the nicest guy. Don't screw it up."

I didn't, and Paul and I married in 1990.

Although my cancer diagnosis felt like one big screwup, Paul helped me push those feelings aside and focus on the goal at hand. Paul was an engineer—an exceedingly patient, compassionate, and thoughtful fixer. He looked at how things worked methodically and carefully whereas I crossed things off the list as fast as possible, always looking ahead, always with a sense of urgency.

He was also an eternal optimist, so conversations about where I'd be buried and how he'd braid Nicole's hair after I died didn't go well with him. I was an unforgiving skeptic and realist who turned to my sister to wallow in how much it all sucked. Paul was my buoy. From his perspective, I would be okay. I would beat this. The more I fought, the more he supported me. The more he was there. I leaned into that optimism and stoic resolve.

For Paul and me, our North Star was a pair of big priorities: doing our best to assure the safety and happiness of our family. And building memories that would last.

Getting to Your Action Plan

You can list your needs and wants, you can place your North Star on your computer screen and note it every day, but how much progress you make is tied directly to your ability to execute those plans. You can't go right from "I have a fatal disease" to "I'm going to keep my family safe and happy." Instead, you must start at one, taking the smaller steps to get you there.

We took the big leap toward pregnancy. Once pregnant, we saw the need for family support to help raise our children. It wasn't fair to leave Paul all on his own living in the Midwest without those closest to him. Moving meant changing jobs, which also meant changing insurance. We prioritized every step, and with Jack's help, we were able to divide and conquer. We did it all with tremendous urgency, still unsure when my disease would become active.

I would feel the same sense of urgency when diagnosed with breast cancer many years later, but for different reasons. No big life changes this time. My goal would be to create as little disruption as possible. Paul had recently started another company but the economy was struggling. He needed to focus if he was going to make this one work. This was not the time to pull out the cancer card.

This time my plan would be to move quickly and put the cancer behind us. Double mastectomy, avoid long-term therapy. I now had *the eight*, a great team of close personal friends that supported me through my myeloma journey and would see me through this one. Cancer would not trump everything this time. Yet somehow it always does. Remember when you make your action plan, things won't always go as designed. Cancer can be humbling. But here are some WTDs to help you take control of the process.

STEP 4: MAKE YOUR ACTION PLAN
WTDs

Start with What, Who, and When
X Establish WHAT you will need

X Identify WHO you will need

X Know WHEN you will need what and who

Break the Plan into Specific Actions

X Get specific

X Get SMART: be Specific, Measurable, Achievable, Relevant, and Time-bound

Recognize Success, Plan for Setbacks

X Celebrate your wins

X Adjust to your setbacks

X Say thank you

WTD 1: Start with the What, Who, and When

With your needs and wants established, it's time to create an action plan that lists the steps you need to take to achieve each objective. While a goal like "not being a burden" sounds like four simple words, it requires us to define what those "burdens" are and the specific what, who, and when it will take to address each one. It also requires us to do something most of us aren't that great at—setting boundaries. You must accept that there are things you may not be able to do. You will have to say no and realize that people are going to have to help you. If you don't let them, it could impact your health both physically and mentally. Here are three initial steps to building your action plan:

✓ *Establish WHAT you will need*

Now that you've broken down your goals into more manageable objectives, you need to identify the resources and support that you will need to achieve each objective. In business, these are called critical success factors (CSFs) and they are essential to achieving your objectives. For example, if your objective is financial security, the CSFs might include creating a budget, reducing unnecessary spending, and increasing savings. You might look at taking out a mortgage or identifying financial assistance programs. Many pharma companies, hospitals, and foundations offer financial aid for patients in need, as well as other services (more on that below).

✓ *Identify WHO you will need*

Just as important as what you need to succeed is who. Who is critical to help you achieve your plan? How can they participate in helping you fulfill your plan? How will it impact them? Is there some sort of middle ground that can work for everyone? You need to identify all the people who can help you achieve your priorities, as well as the people whom your diagnosis directly impacts—spouse, immediate family, friends, employer, colleagues, and so on. You will likely need to depend on some of these people, maybe just a single individual, to execute your plan. They are your partners. Figure out the journey together, celebrate the wins, and always show gratitude for their support.

→ **Lead caregiver**: Start by identifying your lead caregiver, learning their calendar, and syncing it with your appointments. Talk to them about both what you need and, perhaps more importantly, what they need. Tending to someone with an illness comes with its own basket of burdens. You want to be sure these people's needs are not abandoned.

→ **Broader care team**: Think about who else you will need to execute your plan, with an understanding that it may require the support of a partner, a parent, a sibling, a coworker, a child. Even people who are single and don't have an automatic, strong built-in support network can identify someone to be with them on this journey. Not everyone has a family member or unshakable best friend, but everyone has their "one person" who can stand next to you.

→ **Healthcare provider(s)**: Your doctor(s) should also know about your plan and understand your needs and wants, even if they conflict with or add challenges to their ideas and recommendations. Always remember that the American healthcare system's goals are not necessarily aligned with the patient's goals. Medicine's sole objective is to optimize treatment outcomes whereas you may have different wants.

→ **Case/care managers or navigators**: You can also call your hospital, your insurance company, even Medicare, and ask to be introduced to a "case manager" or a "navigator." Patient navigators and case managers are healthcare workers who aim to provide individualized assistance to people facing significant, complex health issues. The terms are often used interchangeably and are described to have overlapping functions, but they are not necessarily the same thing. Patient navigators may be individuals with or without clinical expertise (such as nurses or individuals with lived experience), whose chief role is to guide patients through the healthcare system and help them overcome barriers that prevent them from getting the care they need. Case managers, on the other hand, are usually professionals (nurses or social workers) who focus on the patient's actual care and help them transition between treatments and stages of care effectively. Case management is all about connecting patients with healthcare providers, designing treatment plans, and making sure it all gets done on time—and is cost-effective. (More on this in Part 2.)

→ **Nonprofits**: You may also want to call the nonprofits or foundations to make sure you have the steps right and to see what other resources are available in your area or online. CancerCare, for example, offers counseling with one of their over forty highly trained social workers who each specialize in one area (such as children, men's cancer, women's cancer). And the American Cancer Society offers a twenty-four/seven hotline with access to trained cancer information specialists, fellow patients, and support with rides and lodging. The disease-based nonprofits can provide similar resources fine-tuned for your particular cancer and situation.

✓ *Know WHEN you will need what and who*

Your needs will vary depending on where you are in your journey. And the support and care you need will depend on a schedule neither you nor your caregivers can control. Therefore, it's critical to get as much information as you can, as early as you can, so you can build a calendar with your caregivers.

Start by asking your doctor what you'll need and when. When do I WANT someone to be there? When do I NEED someone to be there? Ask about the timing and needs tied to each procedure. Will I have surgery right away or will there be a watch-and-wait period first? How difficult will that surgery be and how long might the recovery period take? Will there be a window of rest before radiation. If so, how long, and how difficult should I expect the radiation to be? Then make a calendar and share it with your support team. Who can be there when? Who can be a backup if someone can't make it? Make sure they understand that the calendar can change and ask in advance for as much flexibility as possible. I've had procedures postponed for everything from hospital schedule changes to testing positive for COVID. And again, always be grateful for their support.

WTD 2: Break Down the Plan into Specific Actions

✓ *Get specific*

It's not enough to say "I won't be a burden" or "I will be the best cancer mom or dad." Translating broad needs and wants into specific concrete actions will make your plan more achievable. Start by breaking down each need and want into smaller, more manageable actions or steps. For example, if your want is to minimize the burden on your family, an action might be to find health services that are within easy driving distance from your home. Or scheduling appointments around the days your spouse can easily take off. If your want is to spend more time with your children or loved ones, an action would be to work with your doctor to avoid treatment during certain weeks. It's not easy, and there will be times when even the best-laid plans must change on a dime, but it can help. If your want is to optimize quality of life in the short term, your action might be to go for a less aggressive course of treatment with fewer side effects. But if your want is to live longer, you might choose more aggressive treatment, sacrificing short-term quality of life for a chance at longer-term survival.

✓ *Get SMART*

These actions should be specific, measurable, achievable, relevant, and time-bound. There's a business acronym for this: SMART. A specific set of realistic SMART actions can be the best path to achieving your broader needs or wants. And regularly reviewing and adjusting these actions will help you stay on track as you make progress toward your ultimate goals.

WTD 3: Recognize Success, Plan for Setbacks

With the steps in place, you will be able to check the boxes and monitor progress through your journey. It will be important to celebrate along the way what you and your support team will accomplish together, but also be ready for setbacks. Your plan should be reviewed and updated regularly to make sure it still fits your situation and is focused on your North Star. Remember, no plan ever goes as planned. You will need to adapt. Most of all, remember: You're not executing the plan alone. It's important to acknowledge and thank your team every step of the way, whether it's a win or a setback.

✓ *Celebrate your wins*

It's important to celebrate the good moments, no matter how big or small. Making it through surgery or chemotherapy or radiation. Attending a special event. Or just having a good day, going on a nice walk, enjoying a meal with family or friends. It helps you to stay positive and it motivates your support team. It reminds you that you are making progress.

✓ *Adjust to your setbacks*

You are on a roller-coaster ride. To some degree, you have to surrender to whatever happens—illnesses tend to do whatever they want to do. There's only so much you can prepare for in advance and create that safety net. But if you watch and learn, you can adjust to make the peaks and valleys smaller. You will start to understand which appointments you can handle on your own versus those where you need a buddy. You will learn which days you feel too sick to work and which are okay. Adjust your plan accordingly.

✓ *Say thank you*

Whether success or setback, it's important to acknowledge the small moments and to say thank you to everyone involved—from family members and friends to the nurses who are often forgotten. Take the time to put it in writing if you can. Nothing makes a more lasting impression than receiving a sincerely written thank-you letter recognizing your effort. It deepens commitment, motivates them to stay with you, to continue helping.

IN CONVERSATION WITH ARIF KAMAL

Chief Patient Officer of the American Cancer Society

Formally with the Duke Cancer Institute, Arif Kamal, MD, MBA, MHS, is the American Cancer Society's first chief patient officer, or CPO. In this important role, he oversees an eight-hundred-member team focused chiefly on patient needs—providing solutions to the issues that prevent people from accessing high-quality care across the cancer journey, from prevention through survivorship and end-of-life care. As someone who runs an array of navigators who help patients put their plans into action, Dr. Kamal was at the top of my list of experts to approach on the subject.

Q. How do you find the right team to match your desired action plan?

A.   It all begins with your priorities. For example, if you know you can't travel far due to your job or other obligations, your need is a cancer center nearby. Still, you want a high-volume center that can provide all the services for treating your particular type of cancer. If you're willing to travel or hope to get into a clinical trial, find an NCI-designated center. If quality of life is your top priority, think about which hospital or center provides the kinds of services that will address that want, such as meditation, yoga, and nutrition classes. If your insurance only covers certain hospitals, start by calling member services of your health plan and ask which hospitals and doctors they recommend. Then call those referrals. Overall, you're looking for a team that hears you out on all your needs and wants, respects your priorities and plan, and supports you—even if your version of the plan differs from what their ideal "plan" is for you. Make sure you convey your priorities clearly to the doctors and see how well they listen and respect your wishes and values. Many decisions will have to be made during your journey, and you'll take comfort in knowing you've got the right team for you and your plan.

Q. How can patients make sure their action plans stay on track?

A. One of the best, most vital things patients can do is be proactive. Speak up. Learn all you can about the resources available to you. In addition to the medical professionals in your circle, also lean on external resources at places like Cancer.org, Cancer.net, and the NCI's site at Cancer.gov. Call with questions and ask about services that address your priorities. And don't forget to ask about patient navigation, which can further help to execute your plan and stay on track. Patient navigation is increasingly becoming more common in healthcare settings and a key part of our ongoing work at the ACS.

Q. How does one find a navigator?

A. In addition to hospitals, you can find navigators at specific disease foundations and within some health plans. Navigators, who may be nurses, social workers, or lay health workers, can help you match your priorities to your path forward and break through any barriers you encounter. They often know the kinds of doctors you need to speak to and are familiar with the system and all aspects of the journey. As patient navigation programs expand, it's becoming easier to find a navigator that you'll have a lot in common with—someone who shares a similar geographic and demographic profile and may even have a similar cancer experience. The more you have a sense of agency around your care, the better and more confident you will feel going forward.

It's a Boy!

The pregnancy was far from easy, but when David's magical birth came on Cinco de Mayo, 1997, he was the greatest gift to all of us.

Every photograph shows Nicole's joy as she holds him way too tight and Paul's and my relief as we know he is healthy. The intensity of my love for David was boundless. The sense of responsibility that went with that love was boundless, too. The following Sunday, Mother's Day, we went to St. Patrick's, the same sacred space where we lit that candle only ten months before. David and Nicole were with us—David swaddled in my arms, only a week old, Nicole sitting in Paul's lap craning to see over the pews.

Father McNulty's sermon that morning was about mothers—the paths they choose, the journeys they take. It was beautiful. No doubt every mom in the congregation felt like he was talking directly to them—the gift of a good preacher. But I knew he was speaking to me. After he finished, he asked the entire parish to stand as the four of us were brought to the altar for a blessing, our church family offering a prayer for the path we had chosen. It was one of the happiest days of my life, a reprieve from the anguish of having to walk away from everything we had built in the Windy City, our careers, our friends, and our loving community.

Thirty days later we moved to Connecticut. When the moving van pulled into the driveway of our new home, there stood our immediate family waiting to greet us. It was a glorious day, the sun shining brilliantly in a clear blue sky unmarred by clouds. Seeing everyone there—Paul's parents, my mom, Karen with her kids rolling around on the freshly mowed lawn—was a long-needed breath of fresh air, nourishment for a sapped and hungry soul. We felt a deep sense of optimism watching them unload the moving truck. We finished the job in half the time and celebrated with pizza and beer.

That takes me to the third goal of my action plan: building memories that will last. Memories only build over time. Was there a way to buy more time?

One of the first things Karen and I did together in our two-sisters mission to save one sister's life was start a community fund for myeloma research. It began with donations from friends and peers at

Searle, but as word spread to Karen's coworkers, Paul's and my classmates, and Paul's parents' friends, others wanted to help. By the time I arrived in Connecticut, our small fund was already beginning to support much-needed research in myeloma. Karen and I knew it was time to go to the next level and incorporate as a 501c3. I knew this formal "founding" of a nonprofit could be a ton of work and I wondered who would take it over when I became ill. But one big gala led to the "next thing" and our ability to succeed was becoming clear. Less than a year after relocating my family, the Multiple Myeloma Research Foundation (MMRF) was incorporated. There was no turning back.

The long-term goal was obvious: extend life and accelerate cures. The short-term focus was funding research grants to attract new scientists to the field. In the end, the organization would not only help save my life but transform cancer care for millions. The impact on my family was less clear. Clouds were already beginning to eclipse my North Star.

PART 2

Buying Time

Step 5

Get the Right Team

Who Are the Best Players for You?

With your overall game plan in place, now the focus revolves around building the specific team that can best help take you on the journey for the long term—however long that may be. It could be weeks, months, or years.

You want the right medical team, clinicians who will provide the most effective and practical care based on the needs and wants you covered in Steps 3 and 4. You want them to listen to your priorities and take them into account as they work with you. You want them to go to bat for you with the insurance companies, explain your treatment in detail, be clear about treatment risks, side effects, and the days you need someone with you. Remember the importance of the nursing staff and an office that is run efficiently, reachable twenty-four/seven, and provides answers quickly when you need them.

You also want the right personal team, the right person or people who can support your day-to-day caregiving needs and provide practical support like running errands or providing transportation. You'll also want to know who to go to for emotional support, or to be distracted or entertained. It's important to have a trusted advisor, someone who you trust to help make decisions and advocate for you with your doctors or insurance company. Sometimes this will be one person . . . and that's okay. It's not how big your team is that's important, but rather the understanding that you don't need to power through this alone.

Illnesses tend to be wily, selfish, and unpredictable. You want doctors who can work with you through every possibility and pitfall, as well as to have a dependable sideline squad of loved ones who can see you through it all and pick up the unexpected slack when necessary.

New Doctor, New Work, New Friends

We were lucky, settled in our new home in Connecticut near family. We'd found a neighborhood where everyone stopped to talk with each other and welcome us. We'd sought this out intentionally, knowing we wanted other young families around us, other children our kids could play with, other parents to keep a watchful eye, and neighborhood get-togethers.

Although the background noise of my diagnosis never stopped playing, we were still in awe that we had pulled the move off and my lurking cancer had not erupted yet. We felt incredibly grateful having checked off so many boxes in record time; it was a credit to everyone around us. Paul was busy in his new job, traveling a lot, and content even though he'd lost the autonomy of having his own company. But we were lucky that we were able to keep our insurance, and he loved getting to visit his parents frequently. Fortunately for us, they'd lived in the area for decades, they knew all the community hospitals, and as such were able to provide a recommendation for my local care.

Having spoken extensively with Dr. Ken Anderson at Dana-Farber Cancer Institute while seeking second opinions, Paul and I knew he would be my East Coast lead. But it would be impossible to drive three to four hours to Boston for my regular monitoring and future treatments. We needed to find a highly competent local team that could serve as a sounding board with Ken and administer as much care as possible. We wanted to limit the driving and spend every hour with our family. We'd worked so hard to get here. Every day was a gift. We were down to two years.

Nearby Stamford Hospital had a good, well-funded cancer center. On one of my first visits to establish myself as a patient with the right doctor, I had an encounter that would turn into an important lesson. After the usual forms and blood draw, I was led into an exam room where the nurse had already taken my vitals. The doctor sat down calmly, read the records that had been sent weeks ago, and then very, very slowly asked one question after another, as if he hadn't done his homework and had to get himself up to speed with my history . . .

"Let's start from the beginning," he said. "How were you diagnosed? And where else did you go? I see these tests from the Mayo Clinic—why there? And let's see what your bone marrow biopsies showed . . . Okay, and then you had a baby . . . wow, that's something . . . and oh my, you have an identical twin!"

It's all fucking in front of you, I thought. He was writing it all down in slow motion onto some paper file that would never get converted into anything useful or shareable. There were thousands of paper files like mine in endless rolling filing cabinets behind the receptionists.

I asked about stem cell transplants and trials. I pulled out all the articles I'd collected on bisphosphonates and how they inhibit IL-6—a key protein that myeloma cells feed off of.

The doctor knew little about any of this. I was being my typical pushy self, demanding a therapy because I found some early research showing it could help my immune system fight off the myeloma a little longer. He wasn't buying it. But he wasn't the one feeling the urgency of the situation. He said he'd call my doctors and let me know, but was confident that I could just sit and wait—do nothing. *Nothing!* That meant more time, more anxiety, more waiting on the ledge. I was not attuned to his line of thinking; my gut told me to be proactive. To do whatever possible. My gut said to walk away. To disagree with this doctor. If I said anything further, I feared I'd be labeled as a "problem patient." But I was no "sit and wait"-er. I wanted to learn anything and everything that might be happening in the labs or the clinic and anything and everything about my own myeloma. I wanted him to tell me everything new and exciting that I might have missed.

As I left to check out, I ran straight into Lisa, a nurse there who also happened to be friends with my longtime friend Lori. Lori was the first of what would become *the eight*, a group of eight women (including myself) who would be there for each other through endless challenges over the next twenty-five years and beyond. I'd known Lori since I was twenty-one and she was with me in that fateful aerobics class in business school where I'd met Paul. Nurse Lisa (friend-of-Lori) recognized me.

"How'd it go?" she asked, referring to my less-than-satisfying visit with the doctor. I decided to be honest with her.

"I don't feel great about it. He's kind of laid-back. I want a doctor who knows *more* than me, someone who will push for me, for new ideas."

She was quick to respond. "Go up to the desk and ask for Michael Bar. He's type A like you."

"You want me to switch?"

"Absolutely. If you don't click, move on. Never worry about hurting their feelings. They don't mind. He probably didn't like you, either. Do what is right for you. You will be with this doctor for a long time and need to have good chemistry. Dr. Bar is direct, honest, and knows the disease and treatments. He's constantly at the medical meetings."

Like many a people pleaser before me, I felt bad about changing my doctor. I worried I had insulted him when he was probably just fine—it simply wasn't a personality match. I headed to the front desk and asked for an appointment with Dr. Bar. And when I saw him a few weeks later, I was again ready to go in with a few questions:

What is my plan in the short term and the long term?
(Stay healthy, be monitored very closely, and watch where stem cell transplants are going.)
Should I go on an anti-IL-6 drug right away?
(Yes, it can't hurt and may help.)
Are you fine working with Ken Anderson?
(Yes, absolutely.)
How will you communicate?
(You will both get a copy of every test and I will call you the minute I see anything unusual.)

Dr. Bar was prepared, organized, and very happy to work with my lead academic doctor, but also had the confidence to go to battle with anyone when necessary. He had all my test results in his own Excel spreadsheet and told me exactly what I needed to do based on his tracking and studying. This was the bootstrap electronic health record of the day, but it worked. And we were evidently all on the same page—Dr. Bar had the dynamic file, copying both Dr. Anderson and me on it with every test.

Together as a team, we would ride the roller coaster up and down, never consistent, one test result good, one bad, and deciding over and over to hold on while we continued to buy time on the research side. Paul and I drove to see Dr. Anderson every eight weeks for additional testing and to keep learning of any new scientific advancements on his end as well. Knowing a stem cell transplant would likely be part of my plan in the future, we met that clinician and his team as well.

Meanwhile, our kids were an essential distraction. The calendar pages turned swiftly, as David quickly went from rolling over to crawling, walking, talking, and exploring the world. He never sat still, always on the move. A natural-born athlete, with a quick temper and a contagious laugh. As soon as he could hold a ball, one was usually in his hand. He was also smart, with an emotional acuity that instinctively knew what you were thinking before you ever had a chance to voice it, even to yourself. I would come to depend on that in years ahead.

Nicole was also enthralled by her little brother, often right by his side to help. While she was always up for a game of catch, she'd also get him to do what she wanted—making him drive around in her little Barbie car or playing dress-up. She was growing up fast, too—loving preschool and forging new friendships. And even at this young age, she was clearly her Cancer birth sign—sensitive, protective, and loyal. She wanted to be sure everyone was happy around her.

Between my sister and me, there were five kids born within five years, each about a year apart. While Karen and I had not planned it this way, she wanted to be sure and have her children quickly, too, so she could be there when I needed her. Looking back, we could not have asked for a better gift. There is no doubt that the closeness of "the cousins" would get them through many challenges in life. Suffice it to say, every get-together with "the Andrewses" (Karen's family) was a riot of fun and magical mayhem.

Good things were happening at the MMRF as well in these early years. We were growing way faster than expected, funding research and conducting much-needed roundtables on important scientific topics. And while the MMRF's research focus (versus policy or social support) was highly unique back then, it was what I knew from my experience in big pharma. It was my training and comfort zone. And then, in an incredible stroke of serendipity, an old often-maligned drug, thalidomide, showed promise in the myeloma space.

The thalidomide story in the context of myeloma breakthroughs is still talked about today in medical circles. Thalidomide was first marketed as a sedative that caused devastating birth defects and abnormalities and was banned worldwide in the early 1960s. Yet here, decades later, it was showing efficacy in last-resort myeloma patients. In an act of love and desperation, the wife of a myeloma patient conducted her own research to find anything to extend her young husband's life. In a chance discovery, she made the connection that thalidomide might be helpful due to its effects on the formation of blood vessels (among other effects). Dr. Bart Barlogie, a myeloma expert then at the University of Arkansas, worked with her and the FDA to allow the drug to be given to her husband. While thalidomide did not save his life in his late stage of the disease, it showed promise for future patients. I glimpsed sparks of hope. One act of serendipity, followed by intense research and clinical questioning, was making a difference.

People clamored to get into the trials so they could access the drug. The MMRF needed to play an important role working with the drugmaker's parent company, Celgene, and the clinicians running the trials, providing information to patients. The MMRF rapidly became a lifeline, sending out emails and a newsletter, keeping track of where trials were open, and which centers had spots. We were also hearing firsthand from patients how they were doing on the controversial drug—its efficacy and side effects. The phone was constantly ringing. Without realizing it, I didn't just have a start-up foundation out of a desk in our home, I now had a job. And having heard that Celgene was already working on a "safer thalidomide" called lenalidomide, brand name Revlimid, life was going to get busier—in a good way. Reluctantly, I rented a small office in town and hired administrative support. I was determined to see this through. So were the people I'd surrounded myself with. Along with a beautiful family around me, I was making new friendships that I would come to cherish forever.

The eight of us always gave ourselves silly nicknames. When we did galas together it was *Friends for Life*, because that was the name of the gala. When we started getting ready for my transplant, it was *Lunch Bunch*, because while we never used to do lunch (we all worked), now we were meeting on Fridays just to talk and cheer me up. After my transplant it became *Bucket List Buds* so we could do excursions. As time went on, Karen and her kids would simply ask "How are *the eight*?" because the eight of us were always there for one another.

As I mentioned, the first of *the eight* was Lori. She has been my sidekick since we dated roommates after college. I called her after first getting diagnosed because I knew she had such strong feelings about losing her own mother at a young age to cancer. I asked what she wished her mom had done differently and she said, "I wish she had tried harder. I felt like she just gave up. And in a strange way, it made me feel like she didn't love me enough to keep going." Her words have stayed with me since that phone call.

Next to join *the eight* were Tiffany and Elisabeth. We met at a Newcomers meeting. In my past, I never would have gone to a local Newcomers meeting. But Paul and I had new mindsets now and realized how much our family would benefit from a community around us.

Soon after Newcomers, I met Bonnie. She showed up at the kiddie pool, vibrant and full of life—the kind of person with an innate caregiving attitude who wakes up every morning wondering what she can do for everyone else. Bonnie was the master doer. She helped Lori run the auction for the MMRF's first major gala. Together they cranked. At our first encounter, she asked why I'd moved there, and I told her the truth. Her response was priceless: "I am by your side"— and she has been ever since. At my lowest moments, it was always Bonnie who would be there to lift me up and see me through.

Closing the circle were Bridget, Amy, and another great mom also named Lori. When Nicole enrolled in kindergarten, Amy and I became class moms together and Bridget was the master volunteer. We shared classroom duties, loving every field trip from the town library to how to make maple syrup. Lori would go on to serve on the MMRF board for many years.

One by one, my kinship with these seven amazing women grew, as did the relationships between our children and our husbands. Knowing my story, these friends couldn't sit still; they wanted to help. But I honestly felt well enough at this time, and I knew any help I needed down the road as my cancer progressed would come. I wanted to save those chips. *The eight* became avid volunteers for the MMRF, especially at its largest annual fundraiser held nearby every fall. Through their endless hours working on silent auctions, invitations, programs, we all bonded. And their contributions just kept increasing. Before each big event, we would convene in the hotel for a quick drink so I could say thank you. Together, we have shared endless joys and sorrows, triumphs and tribulations.

Building Your Team

For your medical team, it's important to know who you want to call the shots and who you want to take the lead on local execution. You also want to keep the process as efficient as possible. For my myeloma care, I had an exceptional team with Ken as my lead and Michael Bar running execution (and always providing his opinions as well). To this day, I still think this approach is extremely helpful if possible—the combination of an academic lead with local execution from a strong community hospital. I would see Michael every eight weeks for close monitoring and for delivery of my bisphosphonate. I would see Ken every two to three months to get additional testing but also to learn more about the new science and drugs happening in the field. By this time, Ken was building a strong clinical and translational team. His lab became one of the top choices for new pharmaceutical and biotech partnerships. He had his finger on the pulse of cutting-edge new compounds. Our conversations were weekly (sometimes daily) as we discussed my care, but more frequently, how the MMRF could accelerate care for everyone. Ken gave me a window into how valuable oversight from an academic medical center (AMC) can be.

For my personal team, I was lucky that I had Paul, Karen, and *the eight*.

Later, when it was determined I was high risk for breast cancer, I was happy to work with a great team at New York City's Mt. Sinai, an academic center that was a one-hour drive away (assuming no traffic). My initial testing was every six months, so the drive was easily doable during surveillance mode. Yet when we switched to treatment mode, and emergencies came up, visits sometimes became two to three times per week, which was draining. I also struggled to integrate my myeloma doctors at Dana-Farber with my breast cancer surgeons at Mt. Sinai. The systems don't talk easily. I felt in the middle. I learned quickly that heme-oncs stick with their liquid tumors and med-oncs stick with their solid tumors. And plastic surgeons have a different job altogether. Even I failed to ask all the right questions and wish I had pushed harder.

One of the most difficult things I learned during this second bout with cancer was how much strain complications from your physical care can create for your personal team. Nicole and David were scared and did everything they could to help. But they couldn't be there twenty-four/seven, nor would I want them to. Neither could Paul. I was lucky to have Karen and *the eight*. Between all of them, I was always in good hands.

Here are WTDs for building a team with the expertise, compassion, and resilience to see you through your full cancer journey, and beyond.

STEP 5: GET THE RIGHT TEAM
WTDs

Find the Right Medical Team
   X Understand the different types of medical centers
   X Select your lead and hospital

Build Out Your Personal Team
   X Roles of family members
   X Roles of friends

Integrate Your Care
- X Integrate your doctors
- X Integrate the centers
- X Integrate your personal support team
- X Keep all important information in one place to easily distribute

WTD 1: Find the Right Medical Team

✓ *Understand the different types of medical centers*

There are different types of medical centers, each with its own benefits and drawbacks. Understanding which centers are best to treat your specific cancer is critical.

→ **NCI-designated centers**: The National Cancer Institute recognizes medical centers for their rigorous standards and state-of-the-art cancer research. There are more than seventy of these NCI-designated cancer centers, located in thirty-six states and the District of Columbia. They are funded by the NCI to deliver cutting-edge treatments. There are three different kinds:

- X comprehensive cancer centers, which have to meet the highest standards and initiate clinical trials;
- X clinical cancer centers, which conduct clinical research and provide care; and
- X basic laboratory cancer centers, which do not provide patient treatment and instead focus solely on laboratory research.

All NCI-designated centers renew their status every five years with the National Institutes of Health (NIH). Examples of top-ranked centers include Dana-Farber in Boston, Memorial Sloan Kettering in New York, Mayo Clinic Cancer Center in Rochester,

Minnesota, and MD Anderson in Houston, Texas. You can find an NCI-designated cancer center in your region by searching "Find a Cancer Center" at www.cancer.gov.

→ **Academic medical centers (AMCs)**: AMCs contain multiple, distinct layers and are the primary sites for graduate medical education and cutting-edge research (many AMCs are affiliated with a medical school). They are also called teaching hospitals because they work with residents and interns from various medical schools. With physicians, nurses, researchers, and teachers all working in unison at an AMC, patients have better access to the latest medical breakthroughs, resources, and clinical trials at these centers. And many AMCs are conducting bench-to-bedside medicine, meaning they have entire teams of PhD scientists that work in the labs with new ideas and approaches. Those ideas are brought to the clinical community to eventually use at the bedside with patients.

→ **Community hospitals**: Community hospitals are your local hospitals. They won't have the same focus on bench-to-bedside medicine, but they do have their perks and plusses—they are closer geographically, easier to get in and out of, and tend to be friendlier and less intimidating. They may also have contracts with other academic centers. Ask what that partnership truly entails. It may provide access to academic clinicians or clinical trials but it also could be a bit more marketing than true integration.

✓ *Select your lead and hospital*

Decide who leads, who executes. As I mentioned earlier, you really want to have a lead doctor with deep knowledge and hands-on experience in your particular cancer, combined with a strong local hospital that you're comfortable with for ongoing execution. If possible, you want that lead doctor to come from an NCI-designated center or equivalent AMC in cancer. Your local execution can be well served by a community hospital. Here are a few tips to help you choose your team:

→ **Base your decision on the oncologist or hospital**: You may make your hospital selection based on an oncologist you really clicked with. Or you may have decided on a specific center because it is close to home or specializes in your type of cancer, and now you are selecting the oncologist at that center. Either way should be perfectly fine. Just keep asking which clinician sees the most patients like you.

→ **Base your decision on expertise in your cancer and specialties offered**: With over a hundred types of cancer, not every center can excel in each one. Where a patient goes for prostate cancer treatment, for example, can be completely different from a center selected for pancreatic cancer. Sometimes you will see that an AMC has centers of excellence dedicated to specific cancers. Patients with rare tumor types will have to research even harder to identify which hospitals see the most patients and have the most experience (Cancer.net has a landing page dedicated for "Finding Information and Support Resources for Rare Cancers" and includes a list of sites, including links to finding doctors who specialize in a rare cancer).

→ **Become familiar with the resources available to you**: Start with making sure which elements of your treatment can be done there. Do they have a strong surgical team, cutting-edge radiation programs, access to new drugs in clinical trials? Can they support you with a navigator or case manager to help you through the logistics of your care? Do they offer psychosocial support or alternative, complimentary programs like meditation, yoga, acupuncture? If you need help with adapting your diet and exercise regimen to your treatment, do they provide relevant support services? Remember to always ask, and never apologize for asking.

WTD 2: Build Out Your Personal Team

Friends, family members, and other caregivers can play distinct and crucial roles in providing support for your cancer journey. While the specific roles may vary based on individual circumstances and relationships, here are general considerations when thinking about roles and how to build and work with your support team:

✓ *Roles of family members*
- → **Caregiving support**: Family members often take on a primary caregiving role, providing day-to-day support, managing medications, assisting with personal care tasks, and coordinating overall care. They may accompany you to medical appointments and help navigate the healthcare system. It's important to communicate openly with your caregiver(s) and show gratitude (see Step 10).
- → **Emotional support**: Family members can offer unconditional love, understanding, and emotional support. They can provide comfort, reassurance, and a shoulder to lean on during challenging moments. But family members also come with emotional history and sometimes it might feel safer to talk with a friend.
- → **Decision-making and advocacy**: Family members can be helpful in discussing treatment options, making important medical decisions, and advocating for your best interests with your medical team or your insurance.
- → **Long-term support**: Family members can assist in managing finances, coordinating insurance claims, or even exploring supportive care options. They can also help create a supportive environment at home by modifying the living space, ensuring accessibility, and organizing necessary equipment.

✓ *Roles of friends*
→ **Emotional support**: Friends can offer a listening ear, empathy, and emotional encouragement. They can provide a sense of normalcy, a source of distraction, and companionship during difficult times.
→ **Practical support**: Friends, like family, can help with practical tasks such as running errands, cooking meals, providing transportation to appointments, or assisting with childcare.
→ **Distraction and recreation**: Friends can help you relax and enjoy outings or social gatherings that can provide much-needed distraction from the daily challenges of living with cancer.
→ **Advocacy and communication**: A close friend can also act as your advocate, helping to communicate your needs, concerns, and preferences to healthcare professionals. They can attend appointments with you, take notes, ask questions, and ensure that your voice is heard and understood.

WTD 3: Integrate Your Care

✓ *Integrate your doctors*
The healthcare system doesn't make it easy for specialists to talk to each other. They tend to work independently, even when they're in the same hospital. But that doesn't mean you can't encourage their integration. You may need to copy each specialist and be clear about your every step. You want to know, for example, when you are shifting from the surgeon or the transplant clinician back to the medical oncologist or the hematological oncologist.

✓ *Integrate the centers*

This typically means that you're linking the specialist at an AMC with your local doctors, but it can also mean linking two AMCs. If you don't do this integration, mistakes can be made. You also need to know when you shift between the lead AMC and local hospital.

✓ *Integrate your personal support team*

Have open and honest conversations with your potential caregivers about your diagnosis, your treatment plan, and how they can support you. Discuss your expectations and their availability. Keep your team informed about your treatment progress and coordinate schedules when necessary. It's important to establish clear communication channels to keep everyone informed about your needs, your progress, and any changes in your treatment.

✓ *Keep all important information easily distributable and in one place*

Keep all important information in one place that you can easily distribute to your personal support team. Examples include:

→ the hospital location, the wing, the parking
→ the lead doctor's name, location, and phone numbers
→ emergency phone numbers
→ copies of insurance cards
→ legal information like your medical directive and/or a living will and trust

Put every detail in your phone. You can take photos of the most important documents and save those on your phone, too. You will also want to provide these documents to your personal leads.

Provide a schedule based on information from the medical team—biopsy dates, surgery dates, radiation, check-in appointments. Then go to the treatments knowing in advance what you can expect. Will your treatment be delivered orally or intravenously? If it's oral, that's easy, but if it's an infusion, you'll want to know more details. How long does it take? How often will it be performed? Know in advance what you're in for so you can best plan and prepare.

IN CONVERSATION WITH CLIFFORD HUDIS

Chief Executive Officer of the American Society of Clinical Oncology

Clifford Hudis, MD, is a medical oncologist who has watched the evolution of cancer medicine over decades and is famous for his compassionate, empathic bedside manner with patients at top of mind. Today, as CEO of the American Society of Clinical Oncology (ASCO), he's responsible for helping support the prestigious organization's nearly 48,000 physician members so they can provide the best, highest-quality care to their cancer patients. Knowing that this group is so important to the cancer community, yet unknown by many lay patients, I was keen on asking him about their goals and resources.

Q. What should patients know about ASCO?

A. We are unique in that our members are the cancer professionals themselves. About one-third of ASCO's members work in traditional academic centers; one-third work in networks affiliated with the big centers; and one-third are in physician-owned private practices. And some rotate between the big centers and private practices. We like to say we are the voice of the world's cancer physicians, and we strive to build physician networks and relationships. Our goal is to keep cancer doctors of all specialties up to speed with the most current practices and news of research advances so they can best care for people living with cancer and help their patients make well-informed decisions. In addition to our annual meeting, we publish one of the top peer-reviewed journals in oncology, maintain ongoing educational programs for our members, and collaborate with other organizations like the ACS to further our goals and outreach. In fact, our patient-friendly site at Cancer.net is presented in collaboration with the ACS; its prime goal is to speak to patients and their families throughout the cancer journey. We've invested a lot in this site, which has content approved by top oncologists. The site is one of the best ones out there for quality, unbiased information on cancer vetted by top oncologists.

Q. If you were advising a patient on the three things they must do when building their oncology team, what would they be?

A.   First, check to see if your potential lead oncologist is one of our active members. Second, ask how many patients like you are seen on a daily, weekly, and monthly basis. Keep in mind that people receiving care can appropriately value different endpoints and results differently. You want to have a team that respects what you value—and how you want to live as you move through treatment. As an example, quality of life matters more than other treatment benefits for some people in some circumstances. And finally, ask about access to clinical trials. Patients should be biased toward clinical trials, which is where some of the most advanced care is being developed and provided. If you're in a big medical center that has a trial appropriate for you, seriously consider it. This can give you access to a larger number of treatment options than may be available through standard care. And you'll be adding important data to the system to inform future treatments. But you don't necessarily have to be in a big center to access trials. There's a lot of research available at community oncologists' sites, too. In fact, that is an important national effort that we are proud to be helping succeed.

Q. What can patients do to maximize their care if they are getting treated locally but also relying on an AMC?

A.   Integrate your care so you have everyone on your medical team in constant communication and collaboration. You not only want your team within the same hospital to be talking to one another, but you also want your doctors across different hospital systems or centers to be linked. Promoting the interaction between big centers and local clinics can be challenging, and you may be dealing with separate health portals that cannot be synced together in one place online. In addition to asking your primary lead doctor about how best to integrate your care across every health professional on your team, you may be able to find a patient navigator (if you don't already have one) who can help you follow the ideal protocol for total integration. Sometimes oncology social workers can also offer key information and help streamline this process.

❋

Turning Forty

Looking back, I see that these years in my smoldering phase were some of our most beautiful as we balanced family, friends, and the expanding MMRF. Apart from taking bisphosphonates and being closely monitored, my time in doctors' offices was manageable. As much as I tried not to, sometimes I let the anxiety of waiting for test results steal my energy and pull me from the joy around me. Uncertainty is a challenge; waiting with uncertainty even more so.

I passed my fortieth birthday in November 1998, and Paul threw me a party. There were maybe eight couples there and when the cake was served, they asked me to make a speech. I remember telling them how I wrote in my first journal that I needed to live until Nicole was five years old so she would remember me. That was as far as I could get before we were all in tears.

Shortly after that I got a call from Ken Anderson. He called me at home a few days after Paul and I returned from a brief celebratory weekend getaway.

"I saw that your numbers went up," he said. "I already spoke with Michael Bar and know you did, too. I would not worry. It just happens sometimes. We need to see a trend and right now it's just another outlier."

"Okay," I said. "But I'm definitely nervous."

"We'll retest in a month or so."

As we always did, we continued our conversation catching up on our work at the MMRF. With funds beginning to flow, so did the MMRF's influence to convene and attract top scientists. They were following the money and the new science, and we needed them. I was increasingly afforded opportunities to meet and interact with the most accomplished doctors in this field. Ken Anderson ultimately became my scientific lead at the foundation. He chaired our scientific advisory board and worked with me on every major program.

At some point on the call, we shifted to the next International Myeloma Workshop meeting that was being planned in Stockholm the following year and would later become the International Myeloma Society (IMS). We both felt it would be a great place to share our fast-growing efforts and show how much we could benefit researchers with our money and leadership. It would be a place to solicit applications for research grants from doctors with great ideas.

"You should go to that meeting, Kathy, and let everyone know what the MMRF is doing. The progress you and Karen have made in such a short time will inspire these clinicians and researchers," Ken urged me.

"Of course," I said reflexively. But as we began to strategize for our being there, complete with a booth and a research roundtable, something in the back of my mind got me worried. I suddenly realized the conflict. The trip, which would entail several days abroad, would mean missing Nicole's first day of kindergarten. The dates overlapped. *Shit.*

It took me days to think about the trip. How could I miss Nicole's first day? Wasn't this what I'd been working for? What would she think of me? How could I make that up to her? I was torn, but at the same time I knew deep down that I needed to go. In one trip, for a meeting that only happened every two years, we could help convene and fund the best minds in myeloma across the globe. There's power in numbers when it comes to rare cancers. I called my mom to get her input.

"All I ever wanted was enough time to see her off to school," I said to her. "You know that."

"I do," she returned. "Of course I do. But I also know how important this will be for you and your future. Honey, let me take Nicole on her big day," my mother offered. "Don't be disappointed. I'm the perfect substitute. You go . . . you have to go."

Paul, Karen, my longtime friend Lori, and I made the trip that September of 1999. It was weird to be in such a visually striking, bustling old city meeting the myeloma experts from Europe, Australia, Asia, you name it. It may have been a relatively small group versus other medical meetings, but they were a powerful group, laser-focused on one disease—multiple myeloma. We made for a terrific team, each one of us using our skills to make the most of the meeting. Lori leveraged her professional medical sales representative experience while Paul and Karen hustled to make sure we spoke to as many doctors as we could. We cobbled our booth together on a small budget and passed out flyers about the foundation to anyone who'd take them. The goal was to alert medical professionals to our funding power and that we were building collaborations in the field while also building an important direct-to-patient database. My presentation aimed at sharing our progress, articulating clearly our wish to support them and to build speed into the highly fragmented medical system.

In the minutes leading up to my talk toward the end of the conference, I took in the surroundings of all these professionals coming together to solve problems in this one tiny area of medicine that was finally gaining more attention on a worldwide stage. My hands trembled a little as I reviewed my notes moments before taking the stage.

As I walked up to the podium with more than five hundred sets of eyes on me, I pictured Nicole holding my mother's hand tightly as they walked to the bus stop thousands of miles away.

"I am so happy to be here to thank you for your hard work to date, to thank you for the progress we've seen in the presentations over the last few days. Today is our daughter Nicole's first day of kindergarten," I announced. "I desperately wanted to walk her to the bus and wait there with her on this big day. I've thought about it since my diagnosis in 1996. I am standing here now instead because I want to be here for her tomorrow, and next year, and the year after that. I want to be there when she goes to first grade, to middle school, to pick her high school prom dress, and I want to teach her to drive. She has a little brother now, David, who needs his mother, too. Every patient has their eyes on the future. It's how we get out of bed each morning and put our feet on the floor. If we all work together, if we work quickly, we can turn their hopes into reality. Time is of the essence."

We lit a fire at that meeting. The MMRF was already becoming one of the most respected organizations in cancer research. And when I called Nicole afterward, she felt cared for having her grammy come up on this special day to walk her to the bus stop.

Step 6

Get the Right Tests
What Precisely Do I Have?

You now have a team backed by a plan attuned to your wishes. The next goal is knowing as much as you can about your specific disease and your specific biology.

No two patients are alike, even between two people with the same disease. You'll want to be treated in a way that's unique to you and your biology, or what's called the personalized medicine approach. You'll aim to be treated with the right drug(s) at the right time, at the right dose, and for the right duration. That is why proper testing is critical. Diagnostic testing has jumped light-years ahead in the past two decades, and the medical community can now pinpoint with much more precision what you have—and what you can expect. The more you know, the more you stand to gain in time and progress toward your cure.

To achieve the best outcome, you must know which centers offer the most innovative diagnostic approaches. And that entails knowing about those diagnostic keys to begin with so you can ask for them and get them covered by your insurance. No easy feat within our challenging healthcare system.

The Red Igloo Cooler and Precision Medicine

In the years following Stockholm, things continued moving forward with ferocity. I was amazed to watch the speed of science yield new drugs—a reality that should give anyone with a diagnosis hope. Myeloma, a silent cancer for decades, was finally getting its due. And as a medical community, we were working collaboratively to accelerate its recognition on the world stage. Sitting in on many high-science meetings organized by the MMRF gave me early, firsthand news demonstrating how well Thalomid and Revlimid were working; the clinical trials for both drugs were showing promising results. Sol Barer, CEO of Celgene, had become a good friend and a leader committed to myeloma patients. And then there was the entrance of Velcade, the third drug of this trifecta that would revolutionize treatment. Velcade's story commenced in 2000 when I received a call from Julian Adams, a medicinal chemist from MIT who had been relentlessly obsessing over a molecule he'd helped develop and that he believed would dramatically change myeloma therapies. His energy and excitement were undeniable.

"Kathy, this compound is in a phase 1 'all comers' trial to identify the optimal dose," he explained. "The first patient enrolled in this study just happened to be a myeloma patient. And he went into a complete remission. It's incredible and makes sense based on how this drug works."

I was hooked. Very few patients went into a deep remission back then and certainly not in an early trial like this. We moved fast, using an already-scheduled MMRF roundtable organized in a Boston hotel to introduce Julian to an entire team of committed myeloma clinicians and scientists from across the country. In that one meeting, we were able to share his results and frame the trial protocol going forward, investigating in which myeloma patients Velcade would prove most effective. I'll never forget Julian passionately taking over the dinner session to start drafting the details. People who had been scheduled to depart canceled plans and rebooked their flights. Everyone wanted to take part in this historic moment. We shaved months, perhaps years, off the drug development timeline.

Through the MMRF, we expedited the phase 2 study and worked with Adams's team all the way through the FDA's relatively speedy approval. The FDA continued to be a friend to this rare cancer with such high unmet need. To this day the story of Velcade, the brand name of the drug, continues to be an example of success in scientific R&D where the time between bench to bedside is as short as possible to save lives. Years later and now in generic version, Velcade remains part of the myeloma arsenal. And we would come to understand that Velcade was an exceptional option in certain types of myeloma patients. Precision medicine was emerging and would continue to grow.

Working with these researchers only further underscored my drive to track and get smarter about my own disease. I followed my basic blood tests like a hawk. As soon as my blood was drawn, I'd anxiously wait for the first bit of news. The CBC (complete blood count) would show how my red and white blood cells were doing as well as my platelets. We didn't want the cancer cells taking over my healthy marrow and crowding out my good cells. I'd check my creatinine and liver enzymes to make sure they were in the normal range. And I never missed an annual PET scan or bone marrow biopsy—not fun, but critical toward knowing the state of the disease.

Ken was the master of biopsies—the person you wanted at the helm because these procedures can be incredibly painful if not done properly. They require deft, experienced hands to carefully maneuver through delicate tissue and bone to grab the specimen without triggering too much discomfort. Tiny holes are bored into the back of the hip bone to suck up liquid marrow and chip off a tiny sample of spongy bone. The process is quite archaic but can deliver highly prized cells for examination.

When my day came, and as Anderson finished the procedure and began preparing the slides, voices outside the exam room grew louder, closer. I asked what was going on.

"Those are the researchers from upstairs here to collect your sample. They want to get it up to the lab so they can study it in detail," Anderson explained as two young scientists came quietly, practically apprehensively, into the room. They carried with them a boxy little red Igloo cooler. It seemed so crude for something so important. Anderson explained that working on fresh, live cells was a win for anyone in the field—the keys to the kingdom of understanding diseases.

The iconic red Igloo cooler symbolized so much for me. As a transporter of live cells, it may as well have been a transporter of data and potential cures. And it got me thinking. What if we were to collect tissue samples from other myeloma patients? That inspiration led to creating the first and largest multicenter tissue bank ever created for a cancer at the MMRF. But it also got me thinking about my own tissue. And Karen's.

I increasingly ran ideas by Anderson. If studying me was interesting, then what about studying identical twins? Much more interesting. Karen and I lobbied hard to be evaluated together using whatever cutting-edge technology was available at the time. It took months for Anderson to finally agree to study our biological differences down to our DNA's behavior. Karen had no reason to undergo any invasive procedures as a healthy individual and doctors are obviously dissuaded from conducting such experiments on people under the Do No Harm oath. But this was an incredibly unique situation that I would not pass up and Karen was a willing subject who could give informed consent. We were genetically 100 percent the same, so spotting discrepancies could clue us—and the world of medicine—in to my cancer's inner, insidious workings. Where had my DNA gone awry? Which codes were misfiring and feeding rogue cancer cells? Could this information lead to my cure with a targeted, sniper-like therapy? Karen and I were the holy grail of research subjects.

The samples that Anderson and his team retrieved from us went on to be studied for months as they conducted experiments to identify the genes turned on in my cancer cells that were not turned on in Karen's healthy cells. Two years went by, in fact, before the abstract—a summary of key findings—to one particularly illuminating study of us was officially published in 2001 and passed around. Indeed, it takes a tedious amount of time for results to come in, but even much longer for those results to be published so others can glean the new information and potentially benefit. When our genetic comparison finally landed in the office of a well-known Mayo doctor, he picked up the phone and called me. He'd been preparing for the big American Society of Hematology (ASH) meeting that was to be held on the West Coast later that year.

"Kathy, I'm looking at a study of identical twins in this ASH abstract," he explained. This was one of the most respected experts in myeloma research, a doctor who was more of a research scientist than clinician. "One has a deletion thirteen and, more importantly, translocation of four-fourteen. I'm assuming this is you."

He paused, and I let the ensuing silence signal that he had to continue, because I was not following. Abnormalities on chromosome number thirteen, which is one of the twenty-three pairs of chromosomes found in virtually every cell, tend to be common in multiple myeloma patients—that much I knew. But the other intel about some "translocation" or swap of genetic material caught me off guard. He had a hunch the study was about me and my sister, hence the call. And he wanted to chat more about it—to understand what research had been done, and by whom.

I wasn't aware of this paper, which named me simply as a forty-two-year-old female diagnosed with "indolent MM" in 1996. And I had a vague idea about the "four-fourteen" detail, but I asked for more. He kept saying "four-fourteen" over and over again like he'd struck gold. In short, he explained, parts of two different chromosomes had switched places to fuel my cancer. In this case, part of chromosome four had swapped places with chromosome fourteen. Such a rare genomic exchange, which is often written as just "4;14" in the scientific literature, happened to be his area of research, and data gathered from twins could potentially shine a light on some of his hypotheses.

As he worked through his questions, he quietly noted that the changes in my DNA were only seen in a small subset of myeloma patients, about 15 percent of us. To think there was something so interesting about my cancer already circulating in the literature without my knowledge was unnerving. What did it mean? And why was I hearing about this for the first time from one of my Mayo contacts rather than my own treating doctor?

"It's high risk," he said matter-of-factly.

"How high?" I asked.

"One of the toughest."

I heard nothing else after that. The news gutted my Friday night. When he shared that the abstract had been written by the Dana-Farber team with Ken Anderson as the lead author, I knew who to call next. The study had to be about me even though neither my name nor my sister's was anywhere on the document, per patient privacy protocols. I was irked that Dr. Anderson had not brought this to my attention and explained it to me. "One of the toughest" seemed like something I should know. Anderson was seeing other patients in the clinic when I tried to reach him so I left a message, hurled into limbo as I fretted over my fate.

I was already late to pick up Nicole. I rushed out to the car but as I pushed the key into the ignition, I slouched over the wheel and let the tears fall. The day had been perfect, normal, and now one call changed everything. *I should be used to it*, I quietly reminded myself. *I have held my own; I have been the lucky one.* An array of questions zipped through my mind, questions I hadn't thought to ask the Mayo doctor. I had to pull myself together. Another family would be dining with us, adding to the pressure. I wiped away the tears, drove to the sports field and grabbed Nicole, and met everyone at the restaurant, where the conversation flowed; Paul covered for me, keeping the conversation light and quick.

When we got home, I waited until the kids were in bed and tracked down the report's abstract myself. As I read it, I knew exactly where the data came from. I was absorbing cold facts about me that had been siphoned from Karen's and my biopsies from a while ago.

Anderson called me back the next morning—6:30 a.m., at first light. He confirmed that I indeed carried the fatalistic 4;14 mutation. He also confirmed it put me at "high risk."

"Why didn't you tell me?" I probed, trying to control my anger like this was some twisted form of betrayal. It was hard to stay mad at Anderson, who was always the paternal physician who didn't want to raise too many alarms and typically preferred to get more information before making any grim predictions. He assured me that everything would be okay. He brought out his best Mr. Rogers to turn my frustration into a light that would guide me forward.

"Kathy," he said, "this is why you did the tests. This is what we needed to do. Now we know everything about your disease—about your myeloma. It will help you and all myeloma patients. The information gleaned is important for you, for everyone. Let's focus on the progress."

While the news was challenging at the time, he was right. The benefits of sharing patient data were evident later that year when Ken presented the research findings on Karen and me at the annual American Society of Hematology (ASH) conference in San Diego. The ASH meeting is where leading experts in blood diseases including blood cancers come together once a year to share the most recent research in understanding these diseases, and any progress in the search for cures. I went every December for over a decade, missing our wedding anniversary every time.

I was sitting in a front-row seat at the ASH myeloma session. The MMRF typically sponsored this session and Ken was often the chair in this meta-theater of anyone who cared at all about myeloma. At one point, Ken shared a color-coded graphic depicting every characteristic of my myeloma with all its molecular idiosyncrasies—4;14

included. It was the mugshot of my disease, translated into clinical terms. On the same slide, he showed how the knowledge of my disease also provided insights into the current and future targets that the scientists and pharmaceutical companies in the ballroom should care about. While I kept thinking, *Oh shit, that's me*, to myself, I quickly understood how data could spur important conversations and focus the science. Yes, my prognosis was bleak. Yes, the death curves of the 4;14s presented throughout that session made me sweat. But maybe this could accelerate drug development the right way.

The more a company believes an oncology target is real, the more likely they can develop a drug toward it. This balance between conducting valuable testing on patients and using that data to drive drug development remains just as critical today.

Ultimately, my 4;14 example was one of many that would begin to leverage precision medicine. We were just beginning to understand that drug therapies could be combined and custom-tailored to each patient's individual molecular makeup. Precision medicine was already transforming other areas in cancer.

Personalize Your Medicine

I had no idea the value of being an identical twin beyond having my best friend by my side growing up. Once my cancer diagnosis hit, it was clear that having a perfectly matched sibling was the most extraordinary gift. I understood why some patients were envious of my future perfect match for a stem cell transplant. While I was shocked when they said it directly to me, I got it. I really did. But Karen and I truly wanted to give back—not just to our own situation, but to everyone's. We realized identical twins could inform the myeloma space. Why had I gotten this disease and Karen had not? We wanted to be research subjects. We pushed for it.

Looking back and rereading the papers written about us, revisiting Ken's slides of us at untold medical meetings, it's clear that our efforts did pay off. Yes, I was distraught over learning about my high-risk myeloma (especially the way that I did) but knowledge is power and precision diagnostics helped optimize my treatment.

The same would turn out to be true with my breast cancer. Breast cancer is one of the leaders in precision medicine. My biopsy confirmed I was ER-positive (estrogen positive), meaning my cancer cells grew in response to the hormone estrogen and would likely respond to hormone therapy. I was also fortunately negative for the well-known BRCA gene, which is inherited and considered high risk. And while I didn't personally choose a precision medicine treatment, there is no doubt that capturing every bit of data you can at diagnosis and throughout the journey can help save your life. And sharing your data can help save others as well. Keep asking your doctor how you can acquire the best information for your disease and how it can easily be shared with others. Perhaps you can be part of an important patient registry.

Here are WTDs for knowing and accessing the right tests to optimize your cancer journey and outcome.

STEP 6: GET THE RIGHT TESTS

WTDs

Know the Types of Diagnostic Tests

X Basic blood count

X Metabolic panel

X Imaging

X Biomarker testing

X Genomics testing

X Immune profiling

Know Your Baseline, Push for a Precision Approach, Follow Your Trends

X Know the top markers for your disease

X Push for a precision approach

X Follow your trends

X Discuss unusual numbers or trends with your doctor

Make Sure Your Diagnostic Testing Is Covered

X Ask your doctor

X Ask your insurance

X Ask the data-generating companies

WTD 1: Know the Types of Diagnostic Tests

✓ *Basic blood count*

This is a blood test that checks specifically for the cellular components of your blood, such as blood count, hemoglobin (the amount of oxygen in your blood), and platelets (important for blood clotting). If you have a low red blood count (RBC) or a low white blood count (WBC), for example, it could be an indicator of infection, treatment response, or your cancer acting up.

✓ *Metabolic panel*

This is a second kind of blood test that evaluates various sub-stances in your blood such as your blood sugar, electrolytes, blood fats like cholesterol and triglycerides, and so on. It offers a general view of your health status and can indicate problems with certain organs such as your liver and kidneys. Tracking both your metabolic panel and basic blood counts is critical to tracking your health.

✓ *Imaging*

Imaging tests are exactly what they sound like—medical procedures that create detailed images of the inside of your body. These tests are used to help diagnose if you have cancer, assess the extent of the cancer, and monitor the effectiveness of treatment.

Several different types of imaging techniques are used today depending on what you're looking for, how the test works, and how it's delivered.

→ **X-ray**: X-ray is perhaps the most common form of imaging test. It uses high-energy radiation to produce images of inside the body. X-rays are often used to diagnose solid tumors, bone tumors, and other types of cancer.

→ **Computed tomography (CT) scan**: CT scans combine X-rays with computer technology to produce detailed images of the body. It can not only help detect tumors, but determine their size and location, and evaluate the effectiveness of treatment.

→ **Magnetic resonance imaging (MRI)**: MRIs combine radio waves with a powerful magnet to produce detailed images of the body. It is particularly useful for detecting tumors in the brain, spinal cord, and other soft tissues.

→ **Positron emission tomography (PET) scan**: PET scans use small amounts of radioactive material to detect changes in the body's cells and tissues. It can help detect cancer cells in the body and determine the extent of your disease.

→ **Ultrasound**: Ultrasound uses high-frequency sound waves to take pictures of the body's organs and tissues. It is often used to detect tumors in the breast, prostate, and other areas.

→ **Mammography**: Mammography uses low-dose X-rays to create detailed images of breast tissue. Mammography can detect breast cancer early, before a lump can be felt, which can improve the chances of successful treatment. Women should talk to their healthcare provider about when and how often to get a mammogram.

Each imaging test has its own advantages, and the choice of test will depend on the type of cancer suspected, the patient's overall health, and other factors. Sometimes tests can overlap one another or be combined with other tests for a more precise "picture."

✓ Biomarker testing

Biomarkers are increasingly revolutionizing the personalized approach to treatment. Put simply, biomarkers are biological substances that can be measured to indicate the presence of disease. Although the substances tested for a basic panel are technically biomarkers, the term is usually used today in reference to more unique biomarkers in the body that can indicate the presence of disease, such as specific proteins or DNA in a person's blood, urine, or tissue sample. In cancer detection, biomarker testing identifies substances that are produced by cancer cells or by the body in response to cancer. These biomarkers can help detect cancer earlier, monitor the progression of the disease, and assess the effectiveness of treatment.

Not every biomarker test available today is standard but biomarker testing is increasingly revolutionizing diagnostics and treatment today for a variety of diseases. Of all the possible applications, lung cancer has been the poster child for the use of targeted therapies based on biomarkers. A library of biomarkers for lung cancer are now cataloged and can easily be detected with a simple blood test to signify the presence of a specific type of lung cancer. This allows doctors to screen for and diagnose lung cancer as precisely as possible, notably when it can be found early and treated with targeted therapies that match the root defects fueling the cancer. There are several types of biomarkers that can be tested for cancer, including:

→ **Tumor markers**: These are substances produced by cancer cells that can easily be detected through a blood or urine test. Common tumor markers are prostate-specific antigen (PSA) for prostate cancer and CA 125 for ovarian cancer.

→ **Genetic biomarkers**: These are changes in a person's DNA that can increase the risk of cancer or indicate the presence of cancer. Examples include BRCA1 and BRCA2 mutations for breast cancer.

→ **Proteomic biomarkers**: These are proteins that are produced by cancer cells and can be detected in the blood or tissue samples. Examples include HER2 protein for breast cancer.

Biomarker testing is not a perfect tool for cancer detection, and a positive result does not always mean that a person has cancer. However, biomarker testing can be a useful tool in combination with other tests and procedures, such as imaging tests and biopsies, to diagnose and monitor cancer.

✓ *Genomics testing*

As the term implies, this looks at your genetic makeup and can also include sequencing of cancerous cells to determine which mutations are making them cancerous. In general, there are two big types of genomic testing: whole-genome sequencing and genotyping. With whole-genome sequencing ("WGS") you're analyzing the entire genomic DNA of a cell using any one of a number of sequencing methods. There's also something called next-generation sequencing ("NGS") that's like a cousin to WGS—it's a faster and cheaper way to analyze DNA but it doesn't sequence the whole genome. It looks at targeted areas in the genome that can provide certain information. Genotyping is the second big bucket of sequencing technology that aims to look for specific variants in the DNA. It's analyzing specific "rungs on the ladder" of your DNA without sequencing every rung (made up of nucleotides or bases).

✓ *Immune profiling*

Immune profiling is a newer technology that's being used more and more. It's a way to measure the state of your immune system at a given point in time and predict how well you will respond to certain treatments. By knowing more about your immune system, what's working and what isn't, doctors can better understand how therapies, such as immunotherapies, might help activate your own immune system to fight the disease.

WTD 2: Know Your Baseline, Push for a Precision Approach, Follow Your Trends

✓ *Know the top markers for your disease*

With most cancers, there will be key metrics or "numbers" to follow that track the status and progression of the illness. These numbers help you know how you are doing, and whether a certain treatment is working or not. Your clinician can tell you which numbers are ideal to watch through your portal upon routine testing. This allows you to track your progress and know when you may need to raise your hand and ask questions about abnormal results or if something seems awry.

✓ *Push for a precision approach*

In addition to your basic panel and key metrics, you should ask your doctor whether additional testing, such as genomics or immune profiling, can inform a more precision approach to your treatment. Not all doctors include this kind of testing as it's an additional step and might not be part of standard protocol, so you may need to push. See below for information on how to get additional testing covered.

✓ *Follow your trends*

As described in Step 1, your portal is your friend. It contains tremendous amounts of data regarding your disease and can be overwhelming. Still, it is important to go on regularly and see how you are doing. Start with tracking your key numbers and look for any abnormalities. Then look deeper to learn more about your disease. You will also see everything from lab results to the physician notes from your biopsies or scans. If you have any questions, don't hesitate to ask your doctor or nurse practitioner to explain.

✓ *Discuss unusual numbers or trends with your doctor*

Should you come across any results that look abnormal or have been flagged as such (most portals will indicate "high" or "low" for irregular results and give you what the normal range should be), speak up and have that conversation with your doctor. Sometimes, a wonky test result is just that and will normalize the next time you test. Other times, you'll want to take a certain number seriously. Your doctor can help you discern the difference.

WTD 3: Make Sure Your Diagnostic Testing Is Covered

✓ *Ask your doctor*

If you have any doubts about which tests are automatically covered by your insurance and which could be considered "unnecessary" and thereby not covered, start by asking your doctor. You want to be clear about which diagnostic tests your doctor is ordering and what potential other diagnostic tests you might want to consider but may have to ask special permission from your insurance company lest you come out of pocket.

Coverage for some tests might depend on where you live, as is the case with Medicare plans.

✓ Ask your insurance

Next, call your primary health insurance company to ask about which diagnostic tests are covered, and which are not. If there's a test that your doctor thinks you need but is not included in your coverage, ask how you can get it covered. This is also when you'll want to clarify cost issues like your deductible, copay, and maximum payout. Sometimes, things as simple as where you get the test and which type of testing technology is used affect coverage and how much you pay.

✓ Ask the data-generating companies

Companies like Tempus and Foundation Medicine that collect and analyze molecular and clinical data can often help in getting high-tech diagnostic testing paid for if your insurance won't cover it. These companies partner with many of the AMCs and even community hospitals to expand their reach—they want your data because data is important in finding new solutions and treatments. There are programs you can access to ease the financial burden or even remove it entirely. The bottom line: The less you have to stress about money, the more you'll be able to focus on getting better.

IN CONVERSATION WITH ANDREA FERRIS

Chief Executive Officer of LUNGevity

Following the death of her mother to lung cancer in 2008, Andrea quickly became a warrior in early detection research for the disease. Leaving a software company she helped launch, Andrea founded an organization that eventually merged with LUNGevity to become the nation's leading lung cancer–focused nonprofit. I talked to her because they have made great strides in setting the example for biomarker testing and have become a model for other areas in the cancer space.

Q. Lung cancer has achieved so much progress due to testing. How so?

A. Scientists have discovered a number of mutations that drive certain types of lung cancer. These can be identified by biomarkers in the disease, which can be tested for and targeted with therapies including immunotherapies. Lung cancer leads the way when it comes to precision medicine. With comprehensive biomarker testing, you can better determine the best treatment for a patient, including which treatments might not work. We know of at least ten targetable lung cancer biomarkers now that have FDA-approved drugs.

Q. That means patients must get tested for their unique biomarkers so they can better choose treatments. But is this routine?

A. Unfortunately, no. In the ideal world, comprehensive biomarker testing, which has been proven important to select and deselect specific treatments, would be routine. The testing is essential to tell the patient what treatment would be most effective to treat their specific type of lung cancer. This is why we are working hard to fix the disconnect. In lung cancer, science is outpacing how healthcare is delivered and how reimbursements work. Patients need to really push their providers on comprehensive biomarker testing to identify their cancer's unique features that may respond to certain drugs or immunotherapies. A person should know what comprehensive biomarker testing is, know how it is performed, and understand how it is used to determine the best treatments. We have a landing page on our site (LUNGevity.org) that gives you everything you need to know about comprehensive biomarker testing, including a reference flyer you can download to share with healthcare providers and family. We also have a list of questions to ask your healthcare team both before and after biomarker testing is done. Biomarker testing is not only revolutionizing lung cancer, but it will increasingly impact most other forms of cancer to optimize treatment.

Q. How can patients increase their chances of getting these critical tests and having them covered by insurance?
A. Patients need to work with doctors who do this important testing and many have office staff that can help with payors. Over 80 percent of lung cancer care is conducted at community hospitals. Selecting the right one is critical. No matter which kind of cancer you have, find a specialist if you can and connect with other patients like you. For our part, we're working hard to educate patients, their loved ones, and providers about the importance of comprehensive biomarker testing. We are also collaborating with the American Cancer Society to push for the right policy decisions.

It's Time to Tell the Kids

Being there for Nicole's and David's milestones left me thirsty for more. Seeing the science move forward made me cautiously optimistic but also exceptionally eager. Knowing that so many patients were missing out on taking advantage of new science created an urgency I'd never known. I was becoming the most impatient person I knew. I wanted to live, I wanted *more life*, and I wanted everyone else to live, too.

With my mission becoming more public, it was finally time to tell Nicole and David. We'd kept my cancer a secret for years but the kids were finally at an age to bear the weight of the diagnosis. Although they were still young and just barely beginning to grasp the basics of biology in elementary and middle school, I still didn't know how much time I had left. And with more and more people knowing and talking about my condition, and with the MMRF constantly in the press, we were worried the kids might hear about it from a friend. But, more importantly, we were ready. Paul and I were in a much more confident place given the strides forward.

By 2001, we had three new drugs in our toolbox and many scientific papers in publication. This cancer was becoming a model for all of medicine. It showed the power of collaboration among doctors and patients under a single mission. Such a positive state of affairs gave us the confidence to speak candidly about my cancer to Nicole and David, even though they would not fully understand everything right away, especially David, who was all of four.

Paul and I obsessed over how to tell them. We read every book and sought counsel on what to say and how much to share, learning that it's best to do it casually, to avoid too many details, and to address all their questions without answering things they didn't ask. In other words, we were told, act like you're on the witness stand or dealing with the IRS—less is more. I was also told to stress how good I felt, and to mention all the progress with new treatments thanks to the MMRF. Our goal was to be honest without raising doubt, or fear.

We all sat down at the kitchen table; the script Paul and I had written out was burned into our minds.

"Hey guys, Mom and I just need to talk with you about something important for a minute." Once he captured their undivided attention, he asked . . . "Do you know what cancer is?" Paul started.

"Yes," Nicole said quickly. "But I can't explain it." She paused briefly, then asked, "Why, does someone we know have cancer?"

"Yes. Mommy does," Paul said calmly.

Nicole's face fell into a blend of confusion and fear.

"What cancer?" Nicole asked. "What kind?"

"It's called multiple myeloma and it's a blood cancer. But we found it early and I feel really well."

"Will you get sick soon?"

"We honestly don't know. I go to the doctor's every eight weeks with Dad. They monitor me very closely so if/when I get sick, we can treat it."

"How long have you had it?"

"For a number of years. I know you've heard me talk about it for my job, but like many people, you just never made the connection between 'multiple myeloma'—two words you've been hearing forever—and cancer."

The kids knew I worked in healthcare and had heard me talk on the phone with endless patients and doctors about multiple myeloma their entire young lives, but I'd managed to keep the C-word out of conversations. Lucky for me, they'd never tied multiple myeloma to cancer until now.

Our initial conversation was short, but Nicole kept coming back to me with questions throughout the evening.

"Mom, will you be okay?" she asked.

"Yes, honey, I'm doing great, there are new treatments coming out, and I have Aunt Karen's immune system to help me if and when I need it," I said.

"Do other people know?"

"Yes, some people know. Your teachers, for example. I just didn't want to tell you until you were old enough to understand."

"Are there things you can't do? Do you need medicine?"

"I can keep doing everything, and I only need medicine for my bones."

"Can I do the races with you now?" she asked, referring to charity runs for cancer with the MMRF.

"Of course. Just don't beat me."

She would later come into my room with a bag of change from her piggy bank and ask me to give it to the scientists. Pure Nicole.

As for David, whose instinct for comic relief was rooted somewhere in his DNA, his question of the night was the easiest to answer.

"Mom, you got this! Can I have an ice cream sandwich?"

Step 7

Get the Right Treatments
What Is My Optimal
Treatment Plan?

The testing is complete. Now your clinicians have a sense of how to treat you. If you have a solid tumor, you may be planning surgery, radiation, chemo, and/or drug therapy. If you have a liquid tumor, you may also be looking at a stem cell transplant. And there are new targeted and immunotherapies for both. Often you are going to be given a plethora of drugs, some for the disease and others for supportive care—keeping your blood counts stable, for example, avoiding infection, and managing side effects like nausea and pain. You may have to take a watch-and-wait approach, or perhaps you're told to start treatment right away. Maybe a few options are under consideration about when to start, how to start, and which treatments to undergo first, second, third, and so on.

Another question is how are the drugs delivered? If oral, you can take them at home; if by infusion, you go to the clinic or medical center. That means more time, more rides, more scheduling, more stress and disruptions to your life and those around you. You have to keep asking exactly what the master plan looks like. Can it be simplified? How flexible is it? Who is involved? And you must track your progress. Otherwise, how will you know if your treatment is working as expected?

Now is the time to get your calendar back out and make sure you have what you need to get through the process and make room for unexpected detours. Yes, someone on your medical team will map out a very detailed treatment plan for you (be sure to ask them), but remember, there will always be mishaps and changes in plans. The journey has so many trajectories, detours, and sideshows. As it unfolds, it takes more and more from everyone.

My Number Is Up

The watch and wait continued for me until a warm, sunny spring day in 2005. Paul, whose office was just a couple of blocks away, walked into the MMRF office visibly shaken. I caught sight of him through the glass walls across the cubicles when he first entered from the back door. He looked troubled, biting his lip and walking with intensity. Jolted by worry, I thought one of the kids must have gotten hurt. It had been years now of living a somewhat normal life with the cancer at bay. But then I read his face as if I were reading a newly inserted footnote on that message he'd scribbled and left on the kitchen counter in 1996. We knew this was coming. It was always inevitable. After years with "high-risk smoldering" multiple myeloma, the cancer had awakened. The magic show was over.

"What is it?" I asked nervously upon his entry into my small quarters. "What's wrong?"

He sat down and leaned in. "I'm sorry," he said, "but Ken Anderson just called me. He's been trying to reach you. It's not good. Your numbers are way up and it's time to do something."

We called Ken back immediately and he picked up right away. He slowly went through the numbers explaining why he felt it was time to move and recommended another bone marrow biopsy and PET scan to be sure. I looked at Paul squarely, my mind already spinning around what had to happen logistically. First came Nicole and David. They needed to be picked up from school, taken to soccer and baseball, and ferried home again for dinner, homework, and bedtime. This was not the time to tell them. Paul and I wanted to figure out the best plan, gather our confidence, and then share the news when they seemed ready to hear it. It was business as usual.

In a matter of days, Paul and I drove to Dana-Farber to complete the testing. The PET scan, which came back first, confirmed the story: two "spots" we'd been watching on my ribs for years were still there but now there were seven more—some on my spine, too. When you start to light up like a Christmas tree, it's time to go. Fast. The bone marrow results also showed significantly more plasma cells—ugly, aggressive cells, indicative of my cancer's next stage.

The plan was set: I'd first undergo months of "induction therapy" in preparation for a stem cell transplant. By definition, induction therapy refers to the first treatment given in a series to treat a disease, in this case cancer. The induction therapy would reduce the number of cancerous plasma cells in my bone marrow and ultimately prime me for the transplant with Karen's cells. But we had to nail the ideal cocktail of drugs at the correct dosages to get it right without challenging side effects or a poor response. It was a balancing act and why I was grateful to have my team in place and ready. Anderson, who was familiar with all the compounds and had an uncanny ability to think ahead, already knew that the combination of Velcade, Revlimid, and the steroid dexamethasone would serve me best. This option, built on drugs the MMRF helped bring to market, was unprecedented, and I became one of the first patients to receive such an up-front combination.

A few days before I started the induction, I told the kids as I drove them to school in the morning. Ironically, it was about a week after Celgene unblinded their study of Revlimid precisely because the drug was shown to be so effective. Our brief conversation was inspired by the recent positivity.

"Guys," I started. Nicole was riding shotgun and David was in the back seat. Car rides were my favorite place to share news. I had them captive and together. "I want you to know that I'm feeling great . . . but I'm going to finally start treatment. Dr. Anderson says it's time and luckily, some really good new drugs are now available that he knows will help me."

Nicole looked over at me as I continued. I caught sight of David in the rearview mirror as he glanced outside. I could tell he was listening.

"It'll be a combination of drugs," I went on. "We never know exactly how I will react to each one but one in particular, called dexamethasone, might make me look a little funny. And I hear it makes people a little nutty."

"What do you mean?" Nicole asked.

"Well, it might make me a little moodier, my face might swell up, and I might not be able to sleep well at night, but that's nothing new." I paused as Nicole looked out through the windshield in her own thoughts. "So, if I act strangely, it's the drugs—it's not me and it's not you. Okay?" I looked back again at David. He was doing his best to smile, searching for just the right words to cheer me up or make me laugh. "In fact, why don't we have a code word for when you notice anything unusual," I suggested.

"UFO?" David chimed in. We would come to use that code word quite often over the next number of months.

Paul and I traveled back up to Boston to pick up the Revlimid from the center's pharmacy. I was anxious to finally get started. But Revlimid turned out to be more of a challenge than I'd anticipated. No sooner did I begin this incredible oral therapy than I developed a blistering rash on my face and body. It was just a few days into treatment and I was crushed. After all the work we'd done with Celgene to get this drug moving quickly, the one person who was having trouble taking it was me. A WTF moment if there ever was one. My expectations, which had been riding high, were dashed.

It took weeks to make sure it was an allergic reaction and to clear the drug from my body; the next plan was to simply lower the dose and see how I tolerated it. But once more, I hit another bump in the road when my liver enzymes went up. I was put on hold again.

Finally, clean scans of my liver and spleen made for the green light. It was time to go again at a lower dose. And luckily, I tolerated it but after a few months into therapy, my response was not as strong as we'd hoped. Another disappointment. Ken quickly worked with the team to add Velcade, which had been shown in trials to work for patients like me—those who had the challenging 4;14 translocation. And with this trifecta combination, which I tolerated relatively well for about five months, my numbers came down. Now, it was time for that last boost with Cytoxan, the final bomb to my system to clear out any remaining enemy cells.

Cytoxan is a chemotherapy drug. That meant, unlike all the drugs I had taken to date, including the trifecta that was made up of more targeted drugs, Cytoxan would be the one to finally make my hair fall out.

It was a cool, crisp November day. My birthday. *The eight* had taken me for a massage, one last hurrah before the impending transplant. We were all there together. It was a rare and much-needed escape.

"Take a deep breath and try to relax," the message therapist said.

As she worked her way through releasing the many knots in my muscles, I could feel the tension melt away. Between the induction therapy and long workweeks at the MMRF, my stress levels were through the roof.

At the end of my massage, the therapist transitioned to my scalp, applying slow, circular motions with her fingertips. A deep sense of tranquility was washing over me when she suddenly stopped. "I'm sorry." She was holding up a handful of my hair in her fingers.

When I told *the eight* what had happened with my hair, there was a short pause before we all broke into laughter. I don't remember who laughed first, probably Bonnie, who would have instinctively known the right response and wouldn't be afraid to jump in with it.

A few days later, Paul took me to a salon to get my head shaved. It was early on a Saturday morning and Nicole was off at practice. David asked if he could come along and Paul and I agreed, thinking David being there would demystify the process and help take some of the shock away of suddenly seeing Mom bald. Knowing our need for privacy, the incredibly kind stylist, who volunteered her time helping patients like me, opened her doors a bit early and greeted us with a warm smile.

"You tell me when you're ready," she said, with the electric razor in her hand.

"Ready as I'll ever be." I tried to smile as I looked at David.

"I'll start slowly so you get used to it. Do you want to look in the mirror or have me turn you around?"

"It's okay, I'll look."

She started slowly and we all watched the strands tumble to the ground. Then suddenly she was done.

"There," she pronounced. "You have such a beautiful, perfectly shaped head. I know it's hard, but you do look good."

"You do look good, Mom," David echoed as he held my hand and assured me. Paul agreed. To me, my head looked tiny without my hair, emphasizing how frail I was feeling.

"It's just hair," I said with a half-hearted chuckle, surveying my new appearance. We all knew it was a tough moment. I felt like every other survivor when I watched it fall to the floor. I had already bought a beautiful wig with Nicole's advice, but once I got home, the kids voted for me to wear a scarf and ballcap. I ended up buying scarves and caps in every color to match each winter sweater I owned. It would become my uniform for months and months.

Throughout this time, my work leading the MMRF was only growing. Success begets success, and while my wants were telling me to spend these last precious pretransplant months with my family, work needs were taking over. There were patients' lives at stake beyond my own; saying no was not an option (or so I thought). Medical meetings were scheduled years in advance and my role running and/or speaking at those meetings meant traveling instead of staying home. Our work in tissue banking, genomic sequencing, registries, and clinical trials had advanced beyond anyone's expectation, and in record time, but these research programs were costing tens of millions, and I was responsible for raising the money. Our highest-level investors wanted and deserved to hear directly from me. Even with my scarf and ballcap, I would still be the public face of the company—orchestrating galas, walks, and board meetings, and leading Advocacy Days on Capitol Hill. I became the bald, moon-faced woman racing through airports, lifting her heavy luggage into tight airplane compartments, and running on hope trying to feel normal amid the chaos. It was topped off by my need to get it all done before I headed to the transplant.

What truly held our family together during this entire pretransplant period was continuing our annual traditions with the Andrews family. We didn't miss our spring Easter egg hunt in Karen's backyard when my induction therapy was just starting. Or the sports-themed birthday celebrations for the three boys in April and May while dealing with rashes and spiking liver enzymes from not getting the induction cocktail right. Summer was filled with David's baseball games and excursions to Grammy's place as the therapy finally started to work. These routines brought such comfort; we always made sure to keep the memories going. Who would win the mini-golf contest? Who rode the wave the farthest? What are you ordering at 18th Street Restaurant and can we get ice cream after?

The fall brought apple picking at nearby Jones Farms with the crazy corn maze and cider donuts just as I was about to add the hair-shedding Cytoxan booster. Then, head shaved and readying for transplant, the family football game punctuated Thanksgiving and skating at Rockefeller Center followed by lunch at the Olive Garden signaled Christmas. Soon enough, it was January and with our holiday rituals behind us it was finally time for me to enter the transplant phase.

I've never liked the month of January, always so cold and dreary in New England. I picked it for my transplant month (they give you a bit of flexibility) knowing I would be better by spring. So as "go time" emerged, I was ready . . . until my liver enzymes spiked yet again and the transplant date was rescheduled. The delay meant Karen's calendar (and Paul's) was thrown off. Karen had her own therapy to do as part of the prep, getting Neupogen shots to "trick" her bone marrow into overproducing stem cells that she would give to me on transplant day. Fresh cells were always the dream scenario.

On the morning of my admission day, Paul and I kept our good-byes to the kids brief and optimistic. David wasn't feeling well and was lobbying for a "pass" from school (No).

We had never been apart from the kids like this before. They presented me with a beautiful, framed collage of photos from the previous year to remind me how much they would miss me. I told them not to worry and I hugged them tightly.

"I'll be back in no time," I told them. "Aunt Karen and Dad will be there with me. Besides, you'll be so busy with school, your friends, and sports that you won't even notice. And when I get homesick, I'll have this beautiful collage to remind me to get better quickly, and to get home as fast as I can."

"Don't forget to check the website," Nicole reminded me. With Paul's help, she had set up an online destination through Caring-Bridge where she would provide updates on my journey and everyone else could chime in with well wishes and news from friends.

Within minutes of them leaving for school, Paul and I finished packing and hit the road. My mind couldn't help but think about the significance of this moment. We were leaping into the great unknown.

As we pulled out of the driveway, I remarked, "I think that went okay," referring to the kids. "They seem a little worried but—"

"They will be fine," Paul interjected. "I love how David was negotiating to miss school."

"I know, right?" But as I was saying it, I appreciated where David was coming from. School suddenly seemed less important when

Mom was leaving for three weeks to get her immune system completely overhauled.

Karen and Paul had put together a calendar making sure that one of them would be with me the entire time. They would alternate shifts, staying at a nearby hotel so they could get to me quickly and often. Karen was scheduled to stay with me right after the actual transplant so Paul could be home with the kids. We'd also made arrangements with friends to help out with everything from playdates to carpools to meal prep. Thank God for *the eight* and our neighbors.

There was a long segment of silence as we both sat in our thoughts on the drive.

"I'm glad you'll be back home in a couple days," I said. I kept wondering what this extended absence would mean for David and Nicole and felt better knowing Paul was with them.

"The timing will be good," he responded. I knew Paul could use the time to check on his dad. His father was sick as well with late-stage lung cancer, having been exposed to asbestos during his life's work in the chemical industry. He was being treated at the same practice in Stamford as me, with Paul as his lead caregiver. He was not responding to the treatments and had been in and out of Stamford Hospital for months. The two were best friends, and their bond had only strengthened after Paul's mother died from an ALS-type illness just a few years earlier. She'd been diagnosed soon after we'd moved back and lost her ability to walk, talk, and eat. Her mind was still strong but her body just stopped. It was heartbreaking. Paul and his dad took incredible care of her. I did my best to support them. More importantly, I brought Nicole and David by to visit as often as possible. They would jump right onto the wheelchair to give her huge hugs and kisses. Picturing it now reminded me how resilient children can be.

"I know you have a lot going on," I said, breaking the silence. "My cancer blew up at the toughest time. I'm really sorry."

"There's never a good time. I don't mind the extra driving up and back."

More silence.

"Is there anyone else who can help out with your dad?" I asked.

"I have some of his friends coming to visit him. And I'll be sure to keep taking the kids over . . . Let's just get you well and out soon."

"I'm ready."

We were at the hospital's check-in station, back to signing the same endless forms on the same famous clipboards repeating the same information I'd given the center for years. We were then taken to an outpatient area where a resident placed a central line called a port in my chest just above my heart. This was how they'd deliver the chemotherapy and Karen's stem cells. With Paul beside me, I was wheeled up to the small, cheerless hospital room, where an unbelievably kind team of nurses did everything possible to make us comfortable. It was clear they'd watched this scene unfold among many anxious patients and caregivers.

Paul organized what personal items I could have, including my laptop, which would connect me with the kids and anyone following my progress via the CaringBridge site. He replaced a generic landscape print hanging on the wall with the kids' collage. It was the only symbol of life in this isolating box of a room where I'd be the experiment and my cancer cells would be scolded and punished, hopefully beaten back into a remission of sorts. Transplant floors are special places with extra precautions in force for patients who are at their most vulnerable. I would not leave this room for three weeks.

Complications started on day two. My port got infected, necessitating antibiotics right off the bat. One day later came the high-dose chemotherapy called melphalan. Like Cytoxan, melphalan goes after every myeloma cell in your body. These chemotherapy drugs do not discriminate; they basically attack every immune cell. The high-dose melphalan is what makes the transplant so hard. You know your body is going to react, you just have no idea how badly. Then once the melphalan has done its killing, it's time to give you those precious stem cells back. Those stem cells will grow into healthy immune cells that will protect you from this day forward. The transplant regenerates both blood and immune cells.

In some ways, the transplant itself was anticlimactic. The lifesaving infusion simply went through the port in silence and there was nothing to watch unfurl within me. Such a small act with incredible promise. And that's why the doctors and nurses remind you that it is a big deal. As I received this precious piece of my sister on what is called Day Zero, my medical team all sang "Happy Birthday" to the dawn of my refreshed immune system. I quietly celebrate that new birthday, January 23, every year.

Next we waited to see how my body would react to Karen's newly transplanted immune system. While we were identical twins, we had small changes in our genomics that might generate graft versus host (GVH) disease. In GVH, the donated cells view the recipient's cells as a threat and attack them. The result can be dangerous and has to be carefully monitored by the transplant team.

As my donor, Karen had the first caregiver shift while Paul went back home to deal with work, the kids, and all their ongoing activities that didn't stop for cancer. She helped me fight through the nausea with ice chips and distracted me with *Oprah* and *Ellen* on TV. I was getting more tired by the day but holding on.

A few days in, the hurricane hit, just when Karen was passing the baton back to Paul. I descended quickly into a hellacious morass of symptoms as my immune system sputtered through the effects of the transplant. Friendly fire. But it felt like I was on the brink again and at the mercy of my body's inner brawl. The sensations were so intense that it was hard to distinguish between hot and cold, pain and paralysis. In a desperate attempt to get the fever down and manage the GI issues, I lay in diapers on frozen sheets of ice packs with my teeth chattering as the doctors and nurses tried to comfort me. Another angry rash covered my body. I feared the tiniest of movements, not wanting to disrupt any of the machines, tubes, and hands holding sway over my ravaged body. I was totally out of it—the rag doll listening to all the hushed chatter among the nurses and doctors around me doing what they could to keep me settled and safe. Although everyone seemed calm, I sensed their concern.

Because I couldn't bear any light, the room had to be pitch black. And quiet. I lost track of time, to the point that it became a meaningless construct as I drifted in and out of sleep and semiconsciousness. The comings and goings of the nurses and doctors were constant. Ken Anderson dropped in occasionally to check on everything and say I'd be okay. The revolving nurses tried to be discreet and nonintrusive.

Hey, Kathy, I'm just checking your vitals.

I'm here to change this IV . . . this will only take a minute.

Kathy, we're doing everything we can to get this fever down.

In brief moments of lucidity, I thought about how much I missed the kids and how terrifying it would be for them to see me like this. Paul never left my side, holding vigil in the nearby recliner, sitting in the dark all day long. The only moments I truly remember were the ones when I turned just enough to see if he was still there when I felt like I was dying and barely able to breathe.

"I'm still here," Paul quietly said to me. "And I'm not going anywhere. I promise."

I would have lost it if I hadn't seen Paul in that chair to help me. I would have lost it if Karen wasn't home checking on all five cousins and getting them together. The mighty five, as we'd come to call them, could get one another through anything. I would have lost it if my friends weren't keeping things normal as best they could while the battle of my transplant took me down. No matter what you think you know, no matter how much you convince yourself that "you've got this," cancer is humbling.

As I slowly came back to life, Karen returned, and we were cocooned like we were kids again telling stories in a fort we'd built. Although this was far from the playfulness of a makeshift fort, we had good laughs as we did the only thing possible to pass the time: talk.

And hide from everything and everyone else. The hum of the machines droned on in the background. I continued sucking on ice chips, a respite to my dry mouth and fear of the inevitable mouth sores.

"Look at us," Karen said to me from the nearby recliner.

"Is this the darkest hours of our lives?" I returned half-amusingly, knowing full well what Karen was referring to. Her life had bottomed out just weeks earlier, as she went from feeling on top of the world to having a broken marriage, a babysitter who quit, and a serious problem at work that compelled her to resign. Three strikes. And here she was with me, having put everything on hold while bringing me back to life. On some level, perhaps my drama was a distraction, just as her drama was a mental diversion for me. There was plenty to moan and groan about, as well as to find levity in.

"Can I have your husband?" she joked. "Paul has been so amazing. I'd kill to have a husband like that!"

"Can I have your health?" I said. "And that fucking coffee you're drinking?" God, I wished I could have some coffee. Or just one night of sleep without being awakened every two hours.

"What can I get for you? I'll go get something you'll actually eat. Just tell me."

"How about some mac and cheese."

And off she went to hunt down the best mac and cheese in Boston. Of course, by the time she returned I no longer wanted it. The only food I could eat? Pop-Tarts.

Eventually, I had to get myself together. The kids were coming to visit. With Karen's help, I managed to take a shower, change my pajamas, and wrap a colorful scarf around my scalp. It was the same scarf we'd chosen together at Nordstrom back in November after we'd shaved my head.

With Paul right behind them, David and Nicole walked slowly into my room fully masked and gloved to protect me from any sources of infection. The nurses had kindly disconnected me from the IVs so they wouldn't be visually jarring. Still, there was no doubt they were in shock. I looked sick, I was in this sterile room that smelled like antiseptic, and we had little space. They tried to act normal, gently climbing onto my hospital bed with me to carefully give a gentle hug. Together, we opened the get-well cards and watched video recaps of their sports games that I'd missed. David, my distraction maestro, had brought a travel version of Battleship to play, and play we did, cross-legged on the room's bed bench for visitors. Thank goodness Paul knew to keep them moving and promised a great Boston lunch somewhere nearby to get them some relief and get me some rest. As they said goodbye, I so badly just wanted to go with them. I wanted to try and calm them and tell them it would be okay—that I'd get back to "mom" soon. But I wasn't sure myself.

As the days dragged on, the doctors watched my numbers closely looking for signs of my recovery. It was a slow and tedious process, the hours gelling together and the days melting by. By day twenty-one, I was out of my mind and couldn't take the isolation and tight quarters of the transplant floor one minute longer. I begged Ken Anderson to let me go home when, to speed the process, they yanked that port right out. It was Ken's gift to me—hearing my desperation. As we got outside, I felt once again like Dorothy entering Oz, only this time, instead of entering the Emerald City of Mayo Clinic, I was stepping out of her black-and-white space and into the full Technicolor of my post-transplant world. I couldn't believe the feeling of the gentle breeze, the warmth of the sun hitting my face, the sounds of people's voices out and about. On the drive home, my eyes squinted at the blinding and dazzling colors around me. Everything looked electric, bright, and big. It began to overwhelm me. I felt like the smallest thing in the world clamoring to come back to life. At ninety-three pounds I felt too small to work again, too small to face people, too scared to ever, ever go through that again.

"I'm so tiny," I said to Paul. "I wonder if I'll ever go back to who I was. Doing the things I used to do."

"You will," he returned. "It'll take time, but we'll get there."

It's Go Time

Everything we've covered so far is to help prepare you for "go time," whether that's surgery, radiation, chemotherapy, or some other form of treatment that disrupts your life even further. This is usually the most challenging time and can extend for days, weeks, even months. You don't typically have control over the timing but, hopefully, you're feeling prepared as you get started. If you have a good foundation to work from, you can plan well in advance, and the quick-fire issues that surface can be handled with less stress.

Although I survived the transplant, I didn't feel like I aced it. I was sick, frail, and weak; and those three months of "go"—from January to March—were probably one of the toughest periods in my life. And in everyone's lives around me. I was naïve thinking I would be that one myeloma patient who would beat all the stats, the one who would make it out of isolation unscathed in record time. It was not to be the case. As I say, I flunked transplant.

I'm not sure why I had the same naïve thought during my breast cancer journey. I had opted for the double mastectomy. It was an aggressive choice given the early stage of the cancer and the availability of other less-invasive options (yes, they might have worked but they would also require ongoing treatment and no guarantee I wouldn't someday still be facing the same mastectomy or worse). But as my doctor told me at the time, "There is no right treatment, only the right treatment for you." I knew the surgery was not something to be taken lightly, but after stem marrow transplant, I thought I could sail through. Once again, I clearly stated to friends and family that I would be back to my normal self in no time. But also once again, I ran into every roadblock, went down every detour from COVID to surgical infections. I would spend much more time in doctors' offices, hospitals, and emergency rooms than I ever imagined.

It's important to get the right treatment, but it's also important to go into treatment with eyes wide open. Ask detailed questions about the side effects of a drug or the risks of a surgery or radiation before you have them. It's also important to know where the delays will happen most frequently and when things will take more time than anticipated. Knowing every detail helps you plan and helps others plan around you. Here are your WTDs for getting the right treatment for you.

STEP 7: GET THE RIGHT TREATMENTS

WTDs

Know When to Treat

X Indolent disease

X Active disease

X Maintenance

Know What to Treat With

X Core interventions: surgery, radiation

X Therapeutic treatments: chemotherapy, induction therapy, targeted therapy, adjuvant therapy, immunotherapy, cell therapy

X New and novel treatments: follow the medical meetings

X Maintenance therapy and supportive care (including meditation and sleep)

Know How Treatments Are Delivered

X Oral

X Intravenous (IV) injections

X Intramuscular (IM) injections

X Subcutaeous (SC) injections

Know What to Expect

X Plan for physical complications

X Plan for life challenges

X Know how your treatment impacts others

WTD 1: Know When to Treat

While some cancers call for immediate intervention, not all cancers need to be treated immediately. Some, depending on your disease state and personal situation, may not need to be treated at all. Sometimes you want to move fast, but sometimes waiting can buy you time. I know it's counterintuitive, but ideally, you wait for as long as possible and, in that window, new treatments become available. The science moves much faster now, so one year can buy you much more. The key, however, is to obtain exceptional baseline tests as soon as possible when you're initially diagnosed (often before treatment) and to know how often to watch those results. There is a balance to be struck between doing too much testing (especially imaging due to the risks of radiation exposure) and understanding a disease's progression. When thinking about when to treat, it's important to first understand the state of your disease.

✓ *Indolent disease*

This is an inactive disease state that can mean you're in a holding pattern or a watch-and-wait period before requiring more aggressive treatment.

✓ *Active disease*

This is when your disease is progressing and demands treatment of some sort.

✓ *Maintenance*

This is when your disease has retreated or stopped progressing after therapy and you can return to watch and wait, hopefully maintaining this state with or without more treatment.

WTD 2: Know What to Treat With

When it's time to treat, sometimes the treatment choice is simple. Certain treatments are considered "standard of care" by medical experts based on a history of proven outcomes. Other times you may have a choice between a more aggressive or less aggressive therapy. One might have an upside of a potentially better outcome with the downside of higher risk or side effects. Another might be safer and more tolerable but may not yield as complete or curative a result. While made with your doctor, the ultimate decision should be yours, not only based on the science, but guided by your personal needs and wants. In thinking about what to treat, it's important to familiarize yourself with the different kinds of treatment you may be presented with.

Also important is knowing what treatments are covered. The National Comprehensive Cancer Network (NCCN) at www.nccn.org provides the most updated set of clinical practice guidelines for healthcare professionals and patients. This is the basis by which insurance companies, Medicare, and Medicaid determine coverage. In addition to knowing the latest standards of care, it's also important to track new and novel treatments by following the results of key medical meetings related to your cancer. As new treatments become available, ask about coverage for them as well. The different kinds of treatments are as follows:

✓ *Core interventions: surgery, radiation*
  → **Surgery**: Physical removal of cancerous cells, typically solid tumors
  → **Radiation**: Using various forms of high-dose radiation (radiotherapy) to kill cancer cells and shrink tumors

✓ *Therapeutic treatments: chemotherapy, induction therapy, targeted therapy, adjuvant therapy, immunotherapy, cell therapy*
  → **Chemotherapy**: Chemotherapy involves drugs to kill cancer cells or stop them from dividing. Chemotherapy can be

psychosocial, spiritual, and physical. Two areas that are known to be helpful for cancer patients are good sleep hygiene and meditation.

X **Sleep hygiene:** Cancer treatment can be brutal on your sleep, and not sleeping can be brutal on your cancer. Improving sleep is essential for maintaining energy levels, reducing stress, managing pain, and supporting the body's healing and immune functions, which can significantly contribute to recovery. The American Academy of Sleep Medicine (sleepeducation.org) is an excellent resource for good sleep hygiene. Here are a few tips to start:

  X Stick to a consistent sleep schedule, including on weekends and holidays.

  X Make sure your bedroom is quiet, dark, and at a comfortable temperature.

  X Limit screen time on electronic devices before sleep.

  X Avoid heavy meals, caffeine, and excessive alcohol before bedtime.

  X Stay active as physical activity during the day can make falling asleep easier at night.

X **Meditation:** While it is essential to remember that meditation is not a substitute for medical treatment, it can play a supportive role by providing physical, emotional, and psychological benefits including reducing stress, coping with side effects, and improving overall well-being and quality of life. Meditation has even been found to help with pain management and there is evidence to suggest that regular meditation may positively influence the immune system, potentially boosting its effectiveness in fighting cancer cells. Many cancer centers offer meditation programs led by trained professionals specifically tailored to the needs of cancer patients.

WTD 3: Know How Treatments Are Delivered

Your doctor will work with you to decide how your drugs will be delivered. Some drugs may be available in both oral and IV forms. Others might be available in both IV and SC forms. Working together, you may decide that, if an oral drug is available, you would prefer it to avoid more trips to the cancer center along with the concomitant blood draws. In other situations, your doctor might want to keep a closer eye on you for the initial treatments and ask for you to come to the hospital or infusion center. Basically, this decision means knowing what drug is preferred, the availability of delivery options, the convenience factor for the patient, and even how the drug is reimbursed by insurance. Just remember to ask because it will help you to know how long your appointment will be.

✓ *Here are the common methods of delivery:*
→ **Oral**: Includes cancer drugs like small molecules that can be swallowed as tablets, pills, and capsules. They typically have a protective coating that gets dissolved in the stomach.
→ **IV injection**: These injections are usually given by a healthcare professional. IV catheters are typically placed into a vein in the forearm or back of the hand.
→ **IM injection**: These injections are also typically given by a healthcare professional. They are typically placed in the muscle of your thigh, arm, or buttocks.
→ **SC injection**: These injections can be delivered at home and by the patient or caregiver. They are typically delivered where there is subcutaneous fat, such as the lower abdomen, front or outer thighs, upper area of the buttocks, and the outer area of the arm.

WTD 4: Know What to Expect

Before starting cancer therapy, it is important to have a comprehensive discussion with your healthcare team about what to expect and how to prepare. This can range from complications resulting directly from treatment (yes, treatment sometimes makes you sicker before it makes you better) to other unexpected pitfalls, from emotional and psychological challenges to unexpected financial burdens. Also, go in with eyes wide open. As I've mentioned previously, treatment rarely works on a set schedule, let alone your preferred timeline. You can (and should) make a plan, but know that you can never fully anticipate what might get in the way or how long it will take. Let's start with looking at some of the potential complications that can come from treatment:

✓ **_Plan for physical complications_**

Fighting cancer in the body is no easy feat and, as everybody knows, often leads to complications. These may vary depending on the type of treatment, your individual health status, and other factors. Here are some potential complications you should be aware of that could arise during therapy:

→ **Side effects**: Cancer treatments are probably as famous for the side effects they cause as they are for the profound curing effects they often deliver. Side effects can vary depending on the type and extent of your therapy and can sometimes be permanent. You should ask your doctor about the potential side effects of your specific treatment and how to best manage them—and prepare for them. Many side effects can be managed with medication but may still affect your quality of life. Others may be signs of a larger problem, so it's important to communicate any and all side effects to your doctor. Common side effects include:

X   Nausea and vomiting (commonly caused by chemotherapy and radiation therapy)

X   Gastrointestinal side effects such as diarrhea or constipation

X   Anemia (a decrease in red blood cells), which can cause fatigue, weakness, and shortness of breath

X   Neuropathy (damage to nerves), which causes numbness, tingling, or pain in your hands and feet

X   Oral complications, as some treatments can affect your mouth (the lining of your mouth, salivary glands, and teeth) and cause sores and tooth decay

X   Skin reactions such as redness or irritation at the site of radiation treatment

X   Infection: According to a study published in the ASCO *Journal of Clinical Oncology*, "Infectious diseases are the second leading cause of death in the field of oncology. Around 60 percent of deaths are infection related to cancer patients, especially with underlying hematological malignancies." Common signs of infection include fever, pain, swelling, redness, fatigue, nausea, and vomiting. If you suspect that you have an infection, it is important to reach out to your doctor. If left untreated, infections can sometimes lead to serious complications.

→ **Drug-drug interactions**: Some medications interact with one another and can cause serious side effects or adverse reactions. Here are ways to find out about potential drug-drug interactions before you begin treatment:

X   *Ask your doctor:* Provide your doctor and pharmacist with a list of all medications, supplements, and herbs that you are taking. They can review your list and provide guidance on potential interactions, as well as recommend alternative medications if needed.

X   *Research wisely:* Several online resources provide information on drug interactions, such as the National Library of

Medicine's Drug Interaction Checker, Drugs.com, and RxList. com. Just enter the names of medications you are taking for information on potential interactions. You can also go to the drug-specific drug.coms that also list the information.

X   *Read the label:* Medication labels and package inserts are required to include information on any serious potential drug interactions. Be sure to read this information carefully and ask your healthcare provider if you have any questions or concerns.

✓ *Plan for life challenges*

In addition to the physical complications, cancer treatment comes with emotional and lifestyle challenges that can profoundly impact your overall well-being and quality of life. As these concerns come up, you should discuss them with both your medical and personal teams and ask them to provide support and resources to help you get through them. Potential life challenges include:

→ **Depression and anxiety**: Cancer therapy can be emotionally draining and it is not uncommon for patients to experience depression, anxiety, or other mood disorders. If you experience emotional difficulties, ask your doctor to refer you to counseling services or prescribe medication to help manage your symptoms.

→ **Body image**: Some cancer therapies can cause changes in body image, such as hair loss or weight gain (let alone double mastectomy). These changes can be tough to cope with and may affect relationships or self-esteem. Again, talk honestly about how you're feeling. If you're uncomfortable talking with family or friends, your hospital or disease-specific foundation will often provide counseling that is either covered or free of charge.

→ **Fertility issues**: Yes, certain cancer therapies can cause fertility issues or premature menopause. Don't hesitate to discuss these potential side effects with your healthcare team before starting treatment. There may be options for preserving fertility. If your treatment entails a high risk that you'll enter menopause early, you'll want to know that in advance so you're not surprised and can best prepare. The risk depends on the type and amount of treatment you receive, as well as your age. Younger people are less likely to enter early menopause, but don't hesitate to bring this conversation up with your treating physician. It's one of those topics that can easily be swept under the carpet and avoided, but if you're a woman, entering menopause unexpectedly can be alarming and life-changing.

→ **Fatigue and physical limitations**: Simply put, cancer therapy can be exhausting, even debilitating. Carrying out even the easiest of daily activities can become a challenge. You may need to make lifestyle adjustments, such as reducing work hours or seeking assistance with household tasks. Know that it's okay if you can't do everything and be open and up-front with your support team about when and where you need help.

→ **Financial concerns**: Finally, cancer therapy can be expensive, and patients too often face unanticipated financial difficulties from their treatment. Talk to your healthcare provider in advance about any costs and financial concerns. Many providers offer options for financial assistance or support.

✓ *Know how your treatment impacts others*

In addition to the physical and life challenges that you're going through, see if you can also think about how your treatment impacts others and adds to their own challenges. Remember, illness is never a single-person experience. It affects everyone around you who is involved directly and indirectly in your treatment and care. Be aware of that and respectful of their needs, too.

IN CONVERSATION WITH PETER LEBOWITZ

Global Oncology Research and Development Head at Janssen, division of Johnson & Johnson

When it comes to new and innovative therapies for cancer treatment, Johnson & Johnson is on the cutting edge. And it's where Peter Lebowitz, MD, PhD, leads a global oncology team to discover and develop new treatment options. Their commitment to studying multiple myeloma keeps me dialed in to their advancements. They are paving the way for cures across many types of cancers, and I was excited to hear from Dr. Lebowitz about today's treatments.

Q. What should patients know about new treatments?
A.   The science is moving very fast with both (1) targeted therapies and (2) immunotherapies that are revolutionizing treatment. With targeted therapies, you're directly acting on the molecular pathways in cancer cells; with immunotherapies, you're alerting the immune system to attack the cancer often in a very specific way. And both can work in synergy to optimize treatment. Patients today are benefiting from decades of advances in science. In just over ten years, for example, Janssen has delivered thirteen new medicines to treat different cancers and, in some cases, extend the lives of patients. We're not only coming up with novel drugs with innovative approaches, but we're also developing the next drug *regimens* to address paths of tumor escape. Cancer is a complex disease and single drug approaches are not enough if we are aiming for potential cures. With a better understanding of biology, we are now discovering multiple drugs that hit the tumor in different ways. This strategy is only possible because we have developed novel approaches, and these therapies, we believe, can translate into major breakthroughs. It's an exciting time to be in this space. Our mission, in fact, is no longer to "just" develop effective treatments but it is now also about developing what is needed to cure the disease.

Q. Which therapies are most promising?

A.   We are incredibly excited about some of the emerging modalities that make drugs even more precise and effective—especially when they are used in combination. Being able to approach cancer from different angles simultaneously with an array of medicines, we believe, can deliver transformational regimens that truly help patients outpace their cancers. Some of these modalities include small molecules, antibody-based multispecifics, antibody drug conjugates (ADCs), immunotherapies like checkpoint inhibitors, cell therapies such as CAR T, oncolytic viruses, vaccines, and pluripotent stem cells. I can't stress it enough: Patients should do what they can to stay on top of new developments in these promising categories. Be sure to understand the rapid advances in the standard of care and consider enrolling in clinical trials. There's so much out there and much more to come.

Q. What makes for the best outcome in terms of treatment?

A.   As we strive to deliver cures, my five-point essential road map in developing treatments goes like the following. First, leverage the effectiveness of multiple therapies. You often need a combination of highly active drugs, each of which has a different mechanism of action. The sum of those actions is greater than the power of the individual drugs. Second, find drug regimens that work together in synergy or sequentially. Third, have a way to measure clearance of the disease by looking at various metrics including minimal residual disease, or MRD. Fourth, treat for as long as needed until the disease is undetectable. And finally, treat a bit longer to maximize that clearance. Remember, the deeper the remission, typically the better results for the patient.

❄

Back to Life

The house had been deep cleaned in preparation for my return. The kids welcomed me with open arms, nervously hugging me in fear I might break. Only today will they share how my skeletal body scared the heck out of them.

Those first few weeks back home recovering brought me joy and optimism. I threw away everything that reminded me of the transplant—every set of pajamas, every magazine I tried to read, every skin cream with a fragrance I could now only associate with sickness and the hospital. The kids brought every game they owned onto my bed and we played endlessly—puzzles, Yahtzee, Battleship. Nicole made me smoothies while David entertained me with jokes—he could always make me laugh. And thank goodness, the Olympics were on with Bob Costas and Scott Hamilton. I was glued day and night to the TV and the distraction saved me. It also snowed in near-blizzard proportions and I was happy everyone else was stuck inside like me. Nicole and David, always helping, liked to hold my hand and rub my bald head with cream to encourage my hair to grow back. *The eight*, my "friends for life," shared the duties of ferrying in dinners, running errands, and making me laugh out loud with funny emails and wild stories. Although they were forbidden from seeing me in person for a while, they were right there with me.

While my "healing" was taking time, life had to keep going with school and Paul's and my work schedules. Transplant forced me into working remotely long before COVID! Truth is I wasn't ready for normal and didn't know if I could do it. I was still flunking. No A on the test. And I was taking my family down a bit. I wished it was all just done—ring the bell, check the box. But it wasn't.

Despite being relieved and looking forward to "starting over" again, something didn't feel right. My positivity started to sour. I felt down and lost. I felt decidedly caged.

Everything happens for a reason.
Everything always works out in the end.
God never gives us more than we can handle.
God has a plan.
It is what it is.
It could be worse.
There's always a silver lining.
The show must go on . . .

None of those terrible platitudes worked. I was not alone. I later learned that as many as half of transplant patients experience at least one episode of substantial anxiety or depression following release. After all those months of preparing for that one significant event, which had sidelined so much of our actual lives and caused so many other things to fall to the wayside in the interim, suddenly it was over and we were expected to leap back into life at full force. Or at least, I expected to leap. But the transition is not as easy as all that. It's sticky.

"I'm depressed," I told my oncologist. Calling out my depression may have been unusual because most people often find it hard to identify their own feelings and speak up about them, or they avoid doing so because they don't want to take drugs. My earlier work at Merck, however, had given me experience in this arena and I had no problem asking for help. My doctor prescribed medication right away, and my sister got me out of the house, followed by my friend Bonnie.

I started slowly as Karen encouraged me to sit in the driver's seat again and reacquaint myself with the simple task of driving. A week later we went to the most taboo of places for immune-compromised cancer patients—the grocery store. Germs galore. But I craved the confrontation with the pleasures of grocery store life—neatly organized aisles filled with food I'd eat and fresh produce on full display that I could pick on my own. I'd lost so much weight and yearned to taste things I chose.

I called Bonnie and met her in the very back corner of a restaurant in her town where nobody knew me. She could not believe how bad I looked. Then Karen and I even went to the nail salon, another no-no for people like me. But I didn't care. Just having someone massage my hands with cream and warm towels brought me back to humanity. Every new "thing" was a victory, and between the drugs and the gradual "excursions," I was getting better.

But things were not getting better for Paul's father. He deteriorated quickly. Sixty days after my transplant, he was gone. Paul would never be the same. This was his hero, his role model, his truest friend and confidant. He would spend days and days writing the eulogy he hoped would do his father justice. I was forbidden to attend the viewing for health safety reasons but got permission to be at the funeral, where I could only hold Paul's hand and pray he had the strength to get through the service.

Step 8

Know the Right Trial

What Could Be Coming Down the Pike?

You've made it through the tough part—the aggressive treatment. Maybe it was a combination of high-dose chemotherapy and a transplant or surgery and radiation . . . or whatever looked like the biggest hill on the climb thus far. Perhaps you even rang the bell that signifies to all who can hear it that "that part" is over. You are recovering and starting to feel better for the first time in what seems like an eternity. Celebrate this moment. Give yourself some grace. Thank everyone who helped you.

More news will continue to emerge from your medical team. You might learn that they "got it all" during surgery or not. You might learn you are in partial remission or complete remission. This information will help determine your progress, your risk of the disease still being there or potentially coming back.

Over time, a new feeling of anxiousness may begin to brew again. It's normal and to be expected. It's part of the course. Uncertain and wary. What if it returns? What if your markers start to spike again? What if your scans show growth? You can't go through an ordeal like that again. It's all too much.

In the cancer world, we call such a return to the illness state a recurrence or relapse (we'll go with recurrence). You're nervous because you know it gets harder to keep beating the beast back.

This is why it's important to keep yourself in a good place. You want to be monitored closely so if there's a U-turn or any signs of recurrence, they're caught very early and quickly. You also want to become familiar—if you're not already—with clinical trials, which could become key to your survival if the cancer returns. Clinical trials are where novel drugs and treatment protocols are being tested that could be better than standard treatment. Put simply, your next lifeline may come from one of many trials out there that matches your needs. Keeping your finger on the pulse of "what's out there" is an important step in the process.

Trials, Tribulations, and Traditions

A few months out from the transplant, and on the other side of my father-in-law's death, it was time to go through another round of tests to see if the transplant worked. This meant another bone marrow biopsy, more PET scans, and the always anxiety-inducing wait for the results, which finally came in on March 26 as I sat working at my computer at home. Ken sent an email that said it all: "Your results are back. You are in a CR. Congrats!" I had to stop, catch my breath, and read the news twice. I couldn't believe it. I had finally gotten an A on the test. "Complete remission," the famous "CR" term I had seen on all those medical slides during all those myeloma conferences.

I leapt from my chair and ran to David and Nicole, who were doing their homework.

"I got a CR! I got a CR!" I screamed.

They must have thought I had finally lost it. The word "exhilarated" doesn't even begin to describe how I felt. Lucky and rescued. What I'd long thought was unsurvivable had been survived. At least for now. I sent Karen a beautiful bouquet of flowers to thank her and we all celebrated with my favorite treat—coconut cupcakes.

I was wise enough to know that complete remission was not

synonymous with cure. When I called Ken that night, I asked him about my PET scans. Indeed, the two spots still shined bright. We just didn't know if it was myeloma or a remnant from a previous injury. I had fractured my ribs jumping off a diving board at the local pool with David and Nicole (an early warning sign that my myeloma was acting up). Now it was complicating what we were seeing on my scans. What it did tell us was to be cautiously optimistic and stay on maintenance therapy. We both understood that a CR was not necessarily a sustainable cure. Still, a reason to celebrate.

As my hair grew back, the weight came back on and life started returning to a revised kind of normal. It amazed me how busy life can be when adolescents close in on teenagerhood. Nicole would soon be heading to high school and was intensely focused on competitive cheerleading. Tiny, nimble, and steadfast, she was a flyer—the one thrown up in the air in a basket toss. She had no fear. My heart jumped with every launch. The practices and competitions were hours away and we gladly drove wherever the schedule took us. David, now in middle school, was playing soccer, basketball, and baseball, with Paul beginning to relinquish his coaching to the experts. Watching both Nicole and David from the bleachers felt like such a gift. David's complete focus and all-in work ethic was something to behold. No one worked harder than David. And while many laughed at Paul and me for not missing a game, it wasn't out of guilt or obligation; we simply loved doing it together. It was social, "normal," and it took us away from cancer.

I was no longer living in doctors' offices or hospitals. I was back full-time at the MMRF, with renewed energy and optimism about our progress. And now that I could actually go out and do things, *the eight* made sure I did. We started a bucket list of activities, from walking the Brooklyn Bridge and seeing the Statue of Liberty, to our six-mile hikes in Litchfield County. These excursions continue to this day.

But while I was getting back to living, in an unfortunate twist of fate, Karen's life took a turn for the worse. She had gone from warrior mode with me during the transplant to helping me pick up the pieces during my depression. Meanwhile, her marriage had fallen apart and she had no choice but to move toward divorce. The pain showed on her face and her too-skinny body. She was working full-time, commuting into the city, and raising three children, with the oldest, JJ, only eleven years old. She was tired and lost but fully committed to keeping *her* family safe and happy. It made our traditions and memory-making even more important.

Each family event and celebration brought us back to our foundation as mothers. They created a sense of stability in a rocky situation. It didn't matter what adversity was in front of us, Karen and I would create traditions that brought the five cousins together. Family barbecues and whiffle ball tournaments when they were young, mandatory Sunday Fun-day as the kids got older. Even our more formal holiday traditions always looked the same: Thanksgiving football fielded the same teams, Mother's Day brunch at the same restaurant, and Christmas dinner always followed by a whacky $10 gift exchange. It was that "routine" that brought stability when the walls were crumbling around us.

Our mom, the only grandparent alive for all five children, continued to fulfill her role beautifully, becoming another source of support and safety for all of us. During this time, we switched from cancer mode to divorce mode, trying to get everyone through it the best way possible. Looking back at this time, I was so laser-focused on my disease, my family, and the MMRF, I wonder if I gave Karen all the support she needed.

Maintenance Therapy, Recurrence, Repeat

In an effort to hold that M-spike at zero after the transplant, and erase the remaining spots on my PET scan, I stayed on Revlimid (a pill I could take at home), while seeing the doctor every eight weeks for continued monitoring. I was also back at the helm of the MMRF, which meant more days than I would like on the road. The travel and long hours led to respiratory infections that meant I would need to go off the Revlimid until I was better. I often asked Ken if I should just stay off because I kept getting sick; I felt like I was off more than I was on. His response: "There's no data to answer that question."

WTF!

"To be safe, you need to stay on," he kept telling me.

It was another moment where the CEO in me thought: *We can do something about this. The MMRF can build a database that starts to answer these kinds of patients' questions.*

Over the next few years, the organization took on building (and funding) one of the largest and most highly published datasets in cancer. We designed it with open access for any scientist in the field to use, breaking down a huge barrier in the broken healthcare system.

As CEO of the MMRF, I was on speed dial for many patients who were struggling.

"What stage are you?"

"Which drugs have you already been on?"

"Have you already done a transplant?"

"How long was your remission?"

"Where do you live?"

"Can you drive to an academic center?"

"Do you have any other illnesses?"

The new trifecta of drugs followed by a stem cell transplant remained a powerful combination for myeloma patients. But when relapse happened, and it almost always did, the cupboard was bare. We were working urgently with pharmaceutical and biotech companies to find the "next thing," while scouring ClinicalTrials.gov to coach patients on what was out there now. It was no easy feat. A single search on clinicaltrials.gov could bring up fifty trials with endless eligibility criteria not written for patients to understand.

Another WTF!

Over time, we made it a priority at the MMRF to help patients learn about trials with a simpler search engine, emails, and a toll-free number.

It was in 2010, four years from my transplant, when Paul got the call from Ken Anderson again. Ken preferred that Paul relay any negative news to me in person. The blip began when Paul walked briskly into my office with that same determined step and his head lowered. He, too, knew that recurrence was sometimes even harder. He also knew I had used up my options. The cupboard was bare for me, too.

We placed the call to Anderson, who explained he did not like the ugly binucleated cells from my previous bone marrow biopsy. He was not panicking because my other tests looked okay and if this was something, at least we'd caught it early. Together, we looked at every single clinical trial available. Anderson knew most of them because Dana-Farber had since become the top center in myeloma at this point and he was often the principal investigator (the person running the trial). I knew them, too, searching nonstop for patients through the MMRF. We studied what was available in phase 1 or 2 or 3. Having supported many trials at the MMRF, I knew the risks and opportunities of each. It was a balance of getting the best therapy. But I also knew the later-phase trials offered more advantages because the researchers had already figured out the optimal dose and/or combination. I had become an expert in the vast, overwhelming world of clinical trials and regulatory efforts at the FDA.

Unfortunately, our efforts only confirmed what I already knew. I was standing in a desert between treatments I'd already used and ones not yet around. But Ken, functioning as both clinician and researcher, was thinking creatively. He recommended we focus on donor lymphocyte infusion (DLI) where we boosted my immune system with Karen's fresh stem cells again, adding Revlimid at the same time to strengthen the response. This had never been done before. It would be a unique protocol. I would essentially be a "clinical trial of one."

Once again, Karen, Paul, and I headed up to Dana-Farber, where the team harvested Karen's healthy stem cells and gave them back to me in a nonceremonious infusion bag. I took the Revlimid pills alongside the infusion to boost the cells' activity. Because we felt we'd caught this spike so early, we never told Nicole and David, nor the MMRF team or board. It was a relatively easy and uneventful treatment—far from the transplant experience as there was no chemotherapy involved.

Months later, following another bone marrow biopsy, we discovered that it had worked. Still, in the back of my mind, I wondered: *How can we better track my remission? Is there a better, more sensitive way to detect signs of relapse? How can we know if there is even the tiniest handful of lurking cells we still need to get rid of?* I approached Ken for some answers—not just for me, for all patients.

"I talk to patients every day, Ken. One day they're in complete remission, then *bang!*, their M-spike is up and they're desperate. If the M-spike only works so well, is there anything else we can use? Something to catch the myeloma cells the M-spike is missing? Something more sensitive, more precise?"

After a brief pause, Ken said, "There is one test called PCR. It's labor-intensive and not for everyone. But it *could* work for you." PCR (polymerase chain reaction) is a laboratory technology that generates multiple copies of a specific segment of DNA or RNA, making it possible to analyze small amounts of DNA with high precision and sensitivity. "We would have to know the genomic signature of your cancer cells to make it work, but we have that because we did your genomics years ago." This was one more example where the right tests early led to a better result later.

"How do we make this happen?" I pressed on. Ken knew "not possible" was not an answer.

"We would need someone to take this on," he said. "A researcher who knows this space and is willing to commit to following you over time. It would be another clinical trial of one."

And with that Ken brought in one of his researchers, Dr. Kathy Wu. To this day, my mini-trial continues. And once again, the MMRF learned of the importance of understanding the entirely new and critically important field of minimal residual disease (MRD). We would become leaders in this space, too, working with the FDA, academia, and diagnostic companies to pursue early detection assays and diagnostics for patients. If MRD could be routinely tested, if patients knew the true depth of their response, they would know whether to discontinue therapy or be more aggressive. Because of PCR, I was ultimately able to safely go off maintenance therapy and fully get my life back again.

Accessing the Latest Treatments

Clinical trials are a tricky game. The only way to know them is to study them and consistently ask your doctor what might be right for you. But it's a daunting task. Today, only 8 percent of patients are in a trial, mostly because they didn't know one was available for them.[*] And even if one is nearby (often challenging because they are mostly conducted at academic centers), you have to first pass the eligibility criteria and then get to the site often for treatment and testing.

And clinical trials are not always the solution. When it came to my breast cancer, I'd had enough of the fear of relapse and had a definitive option in double mastectomy. My "third opinion," a wonderful clinician at Dana-Farber, said to me, "Kathy, you spent your life helping to cure myeloma. Now you have an opportunity to do surgery and have a 99 percent chance of curing your breast cancer. Take it."

I did. But when I did a quick search for breast cancer trials on

---

[*]   See: Joseph, et al. "Systematic Review and Meta-Analysis of the Magnitude of Structural, Clinical, and Physician and Patient Barriers to Cancer Clinical Trial Participation," *Journal of the National Cancer Institute* 111, no. 3 (March 2019): 245–255.

clinicaltrials.gov, it yielded more than 12,000 studies. How is anyone supposed to figure out which of the 12,000 is the right trial for them, let alone how to get into it? And whether any of these 12,000-plus trials is even an option at all? Here are your WTDs for understanding and navigating trials when a clinical trial might be your best option.

STEP 8: KNOW THE RIGHT TRIAL

WTDs

Know the Types of Trials

X Phases 1 and 2 trials

X Phase 3 trials

X Phase 4 trials

X Investigator-initiated trials

Know Where and How to Find Them

X ClinicalTrials.gov

X Patient and research foundations

X Cancer centers

X Ask your doctor

Know What to Look For

X Trial design and protocols

X Trial location

X Time commitment

X Eligibility criteria

X Making your decision

WTD 1: Know the Types of Trials

Clinical trials are research studies where people volunteer to test new treatments or therapies that may not be available through standard care. The treatment, while still being developed, is free. Often there is additional compensation and expenses are reimbursed. Trials are conducted in phases, based on how far along a treatment is in its development cycle. Each phase of a clinical trial has a specific purpose and participant group. The key phases of cancer trials are as follows:

✓ *Phase 1 and 2 trials*

Trials in phases 1 and 2 are frequently done at academic centers as they require detailed scientific information and can be labor intensive. This is where a potential treatment is tested first for its safety and ideal dosage (phase 1) and whether or not it even works (phase 2). These trials are often started in later-stage patients who have exhausted other treatment options and are willing to take the risk of being in a trial where the dosing and/or efficacy is still being determined.

✓ *Phase 3 trials*

By phase 3, the goal is to compare the new treatment against the current standard of care. Study participants are typically picked randomly ("randomized") to receive either the standard of care or the new therapy. Phase 3 trials may be, but are not always, double-blinded, comparing standard of care with a new therapy. Neither you nor your doctor will know which therapy you're getting. The beauty of phase 3 trials is that they tend to include large numbers of patients, and can be done in many places (around the world) at the same time as opposed to only at academic medical centers. This means you might be able to participate through a local community hospital or doctor's office. If, during a phase 3 trial, the drug being tested demonstrates a statistically and clinically improved benefit over standard of care, all patients are moved to the new drug.

✓ *Phase 4 trials*

By phase 4, which is the safest type of clinical trial, the treatment has been FDA-approved and the study seeks more long-term data on effectiveness, quality of life, and cost issues on a larger and more diverse patient population. Drugs in this phase do not require you to formally participate in the ongoing study—you can still get them. Any compensation or reimbursement is generally much lower in phase 4 trials than it is in phases 1 to 3.

✓ *Investigator-initiated trials*

Investigator-initiated trials are run by nonpharmaceutical researchers working in a healthcare setting and hoping to test a new clinical practice or to compare the effectiveness of existing treatments. They are often designed to answer a question that the pharma company may not have asked.

WTD 2: Know Where and How to Find Them

To find clinical trials in cancer, there are several resources available:

✓ *ClinicalTrials.gov*

This site, spearheaded by the government, is the most frequently searched site for cancer trials. Every trial must "register" its information here and it can be a gold mine for patients. Still, it can be unwieldy and hard to maneuver.

✓ *Patient and research foundations*

→ **Cancer.gov**: NCI offers a custom tool for people to search NCI-supported trials at cancer.gov. You can also talk or chat with an information specialist to help you with your search.

→ **Disease-specific foundations**: Individual foundations often have a robust database of trials with a search engine. The organizations often pull from ClinicalTrials.gov but they curate the information to make it easier for you. In addition, the organization may be able to offer a coordinator or patient navigator to walk you through the process.

✓ *Cancer centers*

Many cancer centers conduct clinical trials and may have information on current trials available on their websites or through patient services. If you're already going to a cancer center, it's worth asking if they have any clinical trials that would be right for you.

✓ *Ask your doctor*

Your doctor or nurse may also have information on clinical trials that may be suitable for you and may help guide you on how to participate.

WTD 3: Know What to Look For

It's important to note that participation in clinical trials is voluntary and involves a serious commitment on behalf of the patient. Here are a few things to think about before committing to be in a clinical trial:

✓ *Trial design and protocols*

A clinical trial "protocol" is basically the blueprint for a trial. It's a detailed document that outlines a trial's design, goals, methods, and procedures. Understanding the trial protocol can help you understand what to expect during the study and make an informed decision about whether to participate.

✓ Trial location

Is the study near you? Is it even feasible to get there? To see this, you must look at the full list of sites included. You may also be able to reach out to the principal investigator running the study. Their clinical coordinator can provide additional information.

✓ Time commitment

Clinical trials involve extensive time commitments. Is the treatment a pill you can take at home or do have to go to the center for an infusion or other procedure? How often do you have to go in for that treatment? How often do you have to go back to the center for testing?

✓ Eligibility criteria

Are you even eligible? Clinical trials have strict eligibility criteria, which could relate to your specific disease, your biology or genetics, your medical history (which you will need to provide), or your age, sex, gender, and ethnic background. Knowing all the inclusion and exclusion details is critical. Most of this will be in a study's protocol, but protocols aren't written for the average person to understand. So look for contact information to find someone who can review a full list of the requirements. Applying for a clinical trial is a detailed process that will involve filling out forms, supplying health records, and coming in for any prequalifying medical tests. It isn't easy, but is worth it if it takes you one step closer to your cure.

✓ Making your decision

Like all treatments, deciding whether to participate in a clinical trial is a personal decision. You need to think about the benefits versus the risks, your current health needs, and, most important, your personal wants. Here are some considerations that may help you make an informed decision:

→ **Benefits and risks**: Before deciding to participate, review the trial's information sheet, which includes details on the potential benefits and risks of participating, as well as the study's goals and procedures.

→ **Be realistic**: Clinical trials can provide early access to treatments before they are available to the public. But it's important to understand going in that not all trials are successful, and some may not provide any benefit.

→ **Ask questions**: You should feel free to ask questions about the trial and discuss any concerns with a trial representative. You may also want to seek support from family members or friends to help you make an informed decision.

→ **Talk to your doctor**: This is a must. Your doctor can help you understand whether a clinical trial is a good option for you and make sure it fits into your overall treatment plan.

IN CONVERSATION WITH MONICA BERTAGNOLLI

Director of the National Cancer Institute

Monica M. Bertagnolli, MD, is a surgical oncologist, cancer researcher, and educator who has dedicated her life to pioneering scientific discovery to improve cancer prevention, early detection, and treatment. Dr. Bertagnolli leads the National Cancer Institute (NCI), the taxpayer-supported federal agency devoted to conducting and supporting cancer research. NCI is the largest funder of cancer research in the world and it coordinates and supports thousands of clinical trials across the country, so she was at the top of my list of people to speak to about these potentially life-saving studies.

Q. What should patients know about clinical trials?
A. Ask about them the moment you're diagnosed so you know what's possible for you should you be eligible to enter one at

some point during your treatment. When I was diagnosed with breast cancer in 2022, one of the first things I asked my doctors was "Is there a study right for me?" And there was. I signed on to it, grateful for all the women before me who participated in trials to arrive at the life-saving treatments I received. The reason you want to ask about trials right away is because some are only open to newly diagnosed patients who have yet to be treated. Don't be intimidated by the fact that trials are studying "experimental" therapies not FDA-approved yet. Some of the most cutting-edge, innovative science is being done in clinical trials—and they are designed to balance potential benefits and risks of being on the experimental treatment with the greater familiarity of being randomized to a conventional treatment. You might receive a life-saving drug that you won't get elsewhere. And the data you add to the research will go on to save other lives. Unfortunately, we don't have enough people participating in trials today, which limits our research and how fast we can find new therapies and potential cures. Part of my goal is to make it possible for everyone who wants to participate in cancer research to have a realistic opportunity to do so, even if you live in a rural area or far from an NCI-designated cancer center.

Q. How do patients find out about trials and know which ones are right for them?

A. Start with your healthcare team. Ask who is up to speed with the latest trials that you could be eligible for. Hopefully someone can step up and provide information, help you do the research, answer questions, interpret the study's protocols, and even push for your inclusion given the eligibility requirements. If you feel that you're not getting the information you need from your team, or your doctors are not knowledgeable about trials appropriate for you, get a second opinion if possible. The NCI can also help. We have a service people can use at 1-800-4-CANCER that's free of charge to provide a tailored search you can then discuss with your doctor. Keep in mind that there are many lists of cancer clinical trials taking place in the US, including on Cancer.gov and on ClinicalTrials.gov, but there may be other trials you want to know about. One could be taking place in your local hospital funded by a drug or biotech company, or even its own researchers. Because there are so many types of sponsors for trials, no single list contains all of them. Also lean on cancer advocacy groups specific to your type of cancer. These groups strive to keep abreast of all the latest advances in research and some can help match you to the right trial that is enrolling patients.

Q. Once a patient finds a potential trial, what should they do to proceed smartly?

A. First, you'll want to know answers to key questions: (1) What is the main purpose of the trial—for example, is it to cure your cancer, lessen side effects, or determine if a potential drug is well-tolerated? (2) How will it logistically work for you? Factor in the logistics of where you need to go, how often, and for how long. Although you won't have to pay to participate in a trial, there are expenses incurred from things like transportation and lodging; some cancer organizations or the sponsoring organization of the trial can help with those costs. These questions are all best addressed by the team running the trial. Ideally, someone on your healthcare team can take the lead and reach out on your behalf, connecting you to a clinical trial team. This gives you and your primary healthcare team the opportunity to learn more and ask questions.

Back to Life, Back to Work

Post-transplant I took incredible solace in that CR. And post-relapse, knowing PCR was monitoring for any signs of MRD, I felt invigorated to move forward with my life and my work at the MMRF. But running a research foundation, I also knew way too much. I knew from the scientists that myeloma was a highly heterogeneous cancer. You would start on one treatment and the cells would mutate and outsmart the therapy. Even in CR you had to constantly look for the next thing. That simple and relentless concern was amplified by patients I spoke with every day. If patients were doing well, they were living their lives and not talking with me. If they were out of options, I got the call. In the back of my mind, I had a sense the disease could always come back. To this day, I will not say I'm cured. I do, however, appreciate the fact that I pursue MRD testing every two to three months at Dana-Farber just to make sure I am being closely monitored. Today, MRD testing is becoming more routine and something patients should continually ask about.

As I read my journals back, I realize how my constant conversations with myeloma patients impacted my work. They were what made the MMRF so extraordinary. I could see every day what patients really needed. I knew firsthand their struggles, their fears, their hopes. It was my window seat into *their* cancer journeys that now motivated me, inspired me, replaced my own cancer as the driving force in my life. We *had* to find new drugs for our relapsed patients. We *needed* to get new clinical trials done quickly and make them much easier to navigate. It was *imperative* that we make data available to everyone for better decision-making. The needs were urgent and demanded immediate attention. Perhaps I should have taken my foot off the pedal. But I didn't.

Shortly after my successful bout with relapse, I would be named one of *Time*'s 100 Most Influential People in the world. I felt more formidable than ever.

PART 3

Living
Ahead

Step 9

Reset (Again)

I Survived, So Now What Do I Want and Need?

Everyone's journey is different. Your disease is different. It may be more or less dire, more or less debilitating. It may be acute, episodic, or chronic—last for years, decades, or the rest of your life. You may be working full-time and your income and benefits are critical to your family. You may be retired and burning through your savings. Regardless, the strength and integrity of your personal support team matters.

Maybe you've relied too much or too little on your family and friends. As difficult as it is, are you truly aware of what else is happening around you? It's never just your worries as a patient. It's what is getting dropped while you and those you love deal with the illness. What did you miss while in the world of active treatment? What did people protect you from while you were fighting the battle? Who was there for you too much? Who was there too little? Somewhere in the liminal space between remission and relapse (or big treatment to less treatment) is time for another "R" and that's to reset.

How is it all going—really? As you enter the period of survivorship, you'll want to rethink, restrategize, and reimagine your life now and for the future. Although it's instinctual to think "it's over" once you've been declared done with treatment (at least for now), there remains a lot to consider. You want to protect the state of your health and future health, but there are also your loved ones to consider. How have your relationships changed? How can they be strengthened? Can you fix what's broken or do you need to move on?

Welcome to this third part of the book that's all about living ahead. To live your best life as a survivor, your planning needs to take a shift. And it starts with the renewed reset of your needs and wants—and relationships.

Trials on the Home Front

It was spring 2012 and everything was blooming, both at home and at work. My MMRF duties were now coming to full fruition. We were busy supporting trials for a promising new immunotherapy drug being developed by Janssen that promised to change the myeloma treatment landscape. The drug, known now as Darzalex, was a monoclonal antibody that targeted a specific protein found on the surface of multiple myeloma cells. By binding to the protein, it would help the immune system recognize and attack the cancer. It would be the beginning of a stream of novel immunotherapy treatments that would create new hope for myeloma patients everywhere *and* hope for me should my own myeloma ever come knocking again. I couldn't help but feel we may actually be able to outright "cure" this disease someday.

Nicole's time in high school was blooming as well. She was now a senior, surrounded by the kindest of friends and a fun, supportive boyfriend. She was cherishing every "last" and so were we. Every competition mattered, every game mattered. When baseball season came around in the final months of spring, she was serving as manager of the varsity baseball team and David was already a pitcher. I did my best to be at every game and to never take work calls, especially when Nicole was cheerleading or when David was pitching. Nicole would drive them both to school every morning and to games on the weekends. I remember smiling in the mornings as they headed out blasting their music, and in the evenings when they'd come back from practice discussing the team and its hopes for the season. This was exactly the scene we'd imagined when Paul and I were working so hard to have David.

Then, just like I pictured during that speech in Stockholm, we were preparing for prom. The little girl whose safety and happiness inspired my entire myeloma journey—from having David to getting my own breakthrough treatment and ultimate CR—was now grown up. Together, we went dress shopping and found the perfect gold shoes and earrings to match. She showed me photos of how she wanted her hair done and we agreed on every meticulous detail with her makeup. The photos Paul took at the preprom get-together reminded us just how happy she was at the time.

To top it off, Nicole had finally received the long-awaited big envelope and was headed to her dream college in Boston. It was everything she hoped for—a great business program, the opportunity to cheer at a D1 level, and the right distance from home.

It was early May and Nicole and I were getting ready to leave for the weekend for college orientation. We were going together while Paul and David stayed back for a baseball tournament. The first event when we got there would be a mass at the school's church and when Nicole came downstairs dressed in jean shorts, I said, "No way you're wearing that to church."

To which she responded, "I absolutely am. Church is only one part of the day."

"You can't. It's disrespectful."

"It's what everyone else will be wearing."

"Please . . ."

"Okay, I will change but still shorts and this is the last time you get to tell me what to wear."

"Good point," I said before adding, "remember to bring a sweater." My mantra because we are both always freezing.

Eye roll but a smile, too.

And I realized my little girl, the one I have written to for seventeen years, the one I have been petrified to leave, was now leaving me. She was not going to be here chatting away about her friends or school, asking what we're having for dinner, deciding which outfit to wear. We are the best of friends. I didn't know everything about her life, but I could read her like a book and she could do the same with me. It was already hitting me how much I was going to miss her.

We drove the familiar route to Boston with her thoughtfully playing music we both liked and we talked.

"I'm glad you're going with me."

"How could I miss your college orientation? It's going to be fun." As I spoke, I heard the irony in my words. I had missed her first day of kindergarten. How many other days had I missed? Not for treatment, but for medical meetings, business meetings, fundraisers.

"Are you ready for your tryouts?" I asked. Nicole had been prepping the necessary stunts and gymnastics to try out for the cheer squad. "You'll do great. Just pretend it's the high school field, not a stadium that holds forty thousand people."

And then we were off to check into her dorm room before heading to mass, where every girl was wearing shorts. I did my best to hold it together when the hymns were sung. She reminded me she is an agnostic going to a Jesuit school. *Do not cry.*

As we went to dinner, I sensed it was a bit like a reunion for many of those around us. We, on the other hand, didn't know a soul. It became painfully apparent when they asked: "How many of you have been on campus before? How many of you are legacies? How many of you are from Massachusetts?" As nearly half the room raised their hands, I realized this would be a new experience for Nicole. I tucked it away in the back of my mind.

As we said good night (the students stayed on campus while the parents found hotels), we had the longest hug and I tried not to embarrass her—*make it quick*. I held my tears until I got to the car and just lost it. *God, this is going to be hard. God, thank you for all the years you've given me with her. Please tell me I've prepared her for this. That I'm prepared, too.*

Before I went to bed, I sent an "I love you" text. Her quick response, as always: "I miss you and I'm homesick."

It was just a few months later when it was time to say goodbye for real, not just for the night or the weekend, but to this entire chapter in our lives I once never thought I would see. We finally drove the overpacked car to her new campus in Boston, getting there two weeks before the other families because indeed, Nicole had made the cheer squad and would be practicing for the first game. It was quiet, with the four of us quickly unpacking the car. And then it was time for Nicole to head to the field. As I would do for years to come, I left a note under her pillow that took hours to write. While it was always easy for me to say "I love you" and share my honest feelings of how much I would miss her, I also wanted her to know how proud she made me, how special she was, and that I was always just a phone call away. Later, when Nicole would use that phone call to tell me how much she was hating school and wanted to leave, I would tell her she could only leave to go to an equal or better college. Did I push too hard? Only time would tell.

Back home, the reality of her absence was potent. I felt so alone standing in her empty room morning after morning, her boxes cleared out, her closet empty, her bed neatly made. Paul was rarely around, having accepted a new position running a small company in northern Connecticut with long hours and a nearly two-hour commute. It was an opportunity he welcomed, but it meant leaving before dawn and not getting home until late. Now I would be the one driving David to high school and practice. I would be the one filling the quiet gaps when he had zero interest in talking at the dinner table. It had always been the four of us, the five of us when you add my cancer. Now with Nicole at college, Paul at work, and my cancer in complete remission, it would be just David and me.

Throughout my cancer journey, David was always the positive one—distracting me with crazy games, making me laugh with laser-sharp quips, or nudging me forward with perfectly timed dares. We had an unspoken connection, with him always there for me, knowing what I needed and when I needed it. Even well into his teens, he would gainfully give up valuable weekends for Mom's annual rituals—apple picking at Jones Farm or skating at Rockefeller Center—cringeworthy for any other sixteen-year-old.

And now was his time to shine. All his hard work and long practices were paying off. He was only a sophomore but already a starting pitcher for his varsity baseball team. But playing varsity baseball meant he was also growing up fast, hanging with juniors and seniors who already had their independence. David was now embracing his own sense of independence, which also meant autonomy from Mom. It was not the best time for me to refocus my energies on him, especially without Nicole or Paul around as a buffer. And let's face it, I wasn't the easiest person. Between dealing with my cancer and the MMRF, I had become demanding on everyone. David would now get the brunt of my fearless intensity.

In short, David's lifestyle took a radical turn as he went from having Nicole drive him everywhere and sharing their wide circle of friendships, to being alone with his mom driving him nuts. I've since tried to erase the memory of helping him practice for his driver's license (which couldn't come fast enough), asking irritating questions at dinner, and nagging him about schoolwork.

One day, as I picked David up from school, I pushed him hard with my concerns about friends, partying, grades, you name it. His every move loomed large under the peering lens of my new laser spotlight. I felt like we were out of runway with his high school years flying by and college applications on the horizon. When he got home, he proceeded to dump his backpack in his room, walk through the kitchen, and state: "I've had enough. You're in my grill. Just please back off." And with that, he walked out the front door. At nearly six feet tall, there was no way I could stop him. I texted. No response. Again. Still no response. Fortunately, I knew that he was coaching a team of young ballplayers and they had practice later that evening. Even in his toughest moments, David was responsible and wouldn't let those kids down. My hunch was he would walk to that practice and be there for them. I waited in the parking lot and when practice was over texted "I'm sorry. Please get in the damn car." He did.

His growing independence was bound to reach a critical juncture. And indeed, it all culminated in a party David threw at our house, which was under renovation at the time. We were living in a rental five minutes away. The local police ended up at the front door; Paul and I got the call and raced over. David was immediately suspended from the team for a number of games. This is when I realized I needed to do something. We had been on one trajectory his entire life, now both our individual needs and wants were shifting, and we hadn't set any framework to accommodate them. We needed . . . I *needed* another personal reset.

My first call was to my friend Tiffany (one of *the eight*). She knew what it was like to raise boys having raised three herself, one Nicole's age and twins that were David's age. She'd known David since he was a baby at Newcomers and was always a great source for kid talk, especially now as the kids were embracing teenage independence. She was a huge help. She gave me perspective on where I should draw the line and where I shouldn't (though I'm not sure David would agree). And because her twin boys were friends with David at school (they are still friends to this day), she was also able to give me a window into David that I couldn't see.

Next, I reached out to both his coach and school counselor for advice. His coach, Mitch Hoffman, whom he respected greatly, reminded me what a tough age David was at and warned David how much talent he was giving up by making these kinds of mistakes. His counselor advised me to ask three questions: "Why did you throw the party? What is it that you dream of? How can we help get you there?"

What a beautiful set of questions. No judgment, simply support. David answered them clearly and in his usual direct way.

Why'd you throw the party? "It was my turn to throw a party; we all take turns."

What do you dream of? "To play baseball in college."

How can we help? "Find the right schools."

Typical David. Straightforward and honest. Kind of funny . . . and yet not.

My last piece of advice came during a lunch meeting with a dear friend and colleague, Lee. It was also my most important piece of advice because it was about me, not David.

I shared what I was feeling about how my relationship with David was becoming unmoored.

"You put way too much work into your work," she said. "It's time to put your family first."

She was telling me the same thing *the eight* said every time they tried to schedule get-togethers with me. "You work way too hard. You live on the road way too much. We're worried about you."

"Go home right now and tell your board chair you need to make some changes," she continued. "Just do it now. Say it out loud. Yes, you're late. Yes, you should have been better focused, but you still have time."

I took her words seriously. That afternoon, I called our chairman. Together, we discussed ways to provide me more flexibility and support. My new role gave me more time to be home and present. David would never want me micromanaging him, but at least he'd know how much I cared and that his dreams were mine as well. We started by making a pact that sits in my top desk drawer to this day. It's a contract on a blank piece of paper stating our expectations of each other. He needed to attain and maintain B grades, get to the key college tournaments (five were listed), and never miss school. In return, I would give him space and privacy. I would trust him to make better decisions. And though I didn't articulate my pledge to be more present at home and less consumed by work, that was surely part of the bargain.

The Other Side

As you get through "the worst of it," the most challenging part of your treatment, all you can focus on is surviving. As you gradually come out on the other side, you know it's time for everyone who helped you to get back to their own lives. It's also time for you to get back to "life." But it's not always that easy. You feel different because you are different and your needs and wants have changed both physically and emotionally. It has been a battle. You see the scars. It's time to face the beauty and the destruction. What's better now? What's worse? What can you do to turn anything bad into good? Where is your North Star now? Most important: Whose needs and wants have changed *other than your own*? And how can you accommodate those now?

My myeloma journey was long. My family had been through the highs and lows while the kids were growing and my sister was struggling. And all the while I was working tirelessly to find new drugs and generate data to save my life and everyone else's. Saving my life took over living my life. I missed the signals.

Paul was looking for calm and to get back the career he put on hold. Nicole was needing my support while at college. Karen needed a friend and confidante. David was just hoping college would get him a break from my pushing. And my friends, well, they just missed me. Nobody was looking me directly in the eye and telling me where I'd gone wrong or where I'd gone absent. People just don't do that to cancer patients. Instead, thoughts are left unsaid. Resentment builds.

Going through breast cancer, it would become clear where I had done the reset right and where I was still missing the signals. I was well aware the sacrifices my family had made in my myeloma days and didn't want to risk harming those relationships again in any way. I had drawn every bit of support I could from them and I wanted to replenish what I had spent, not take more. The double mastectomy was supposed to get me off the roller coaster quickly so I could do just that. But again, it was not to be. A one-and-done procedure turned into endless infections and more surgery. I was in and out of hospitals and ERs for eighteen months. It took a toll all over again. On me, on them, on everyone.

As you rethink your life and relationships post-treatment, remember that personal resets are not one-and-done, either. Here are your WTDs for living ahead.

STEP 9: RESET (AGAIN)

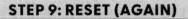

WTDs

Reset Your Needs
   X Physical needs
   X Emotional needs
   X Financial needs

Reset Your Wants
   X Revisit your "North Star"
   X Commit, sign, and post . . . again!

Reset Your Relationships
   X Recognize the damage caused
   X Have the difficult conversations

WTD 1: Reset Your Needs

✓ *Physical needs*

There's no doubt you are looking at your body in a new way. You may be seeing the scars from surgery, feeling the fatigue from chemotherapy or general pain from the overall experience. What can you do to start building yourself back up? It might be simple walks outside or becoming more active with your children, family, and friends. It might be checking off things on your own bucket list, excursions you missed during treatment or adventures you never thought you would have. At this point, you are still seeing a physician who can walk you through the appropriate follow-up plan for your specific cancer. The doctor you're seeing is likely the medical oncologist or hematologist-oncologist you've worked with from the beginning. Sometimes patients are also referred to their primary care doctor. Once you know the plan, check your coverage to see if you have access to physical therapy or occupational therapy. See if your hospital offers or recommends other wellness programs you can do alone or with others. This can help get you back to "normal" more quickly.

✓ *Emotional needs*

It is common for survivors to feel grateful once they are through the treatment. They might be looking at cancer as a positive, something that helped them realize how precious time can be. But it's also common to feel anxiety and depression. You may also feel stressed that the cancer may come back and you can't handle it again. This is the time to speak with your doctor and, again, ask for a care plan. You have options—from support groups to counseling to medication.

✓ *Financial needs*

As previously mentioned, financial toxicity is a real thing for cancer patients and their families. You may have lost significant time at work, you may have lost insurance, and you may not be sure when you can get back to a full-time job. This is the time to reach out to the billing office at your requisite center and your doctors' offices. Start to understand the types of payment plans they offer. Also ask them to help you dispute bills that were not covered with the insurance company and/or Medicare and Medicaid. It can be exhausting but it's worth it. The billing offices in the hospitals know how to help you fight this battle. Work with them.

WTD 2: Reset Your Wants

Life has changed and you've learned a lot. Clearly, you know the importance of your health. But there's more, much more, to living ahead than simply preparing for the possible worst.

✓ *Revisit your "North Star"*

Are the wants you established back in Step 3 still the most important? Have you identified new ones?

Would you change the balance between work and home? Would you change how you want to spend your time? Who you want to spend it with? It's time to start with a new blank sheet of paper. Go back to Step 3 and rethink what really matters now, then write it down.

✓ *Commit, sign, and post . . . again!*

Place your new wants where you can see them every day. Life will start moving fast. You won't get this time back to do this important bit of reflection.

WTD 3: Reset Your Relationships

Kate Bowler, author of *No Cure for Being Human*, and Suleika Jaouad, author of *Between Two Kingdoms*, share beautiful wisdom on the cancer journey and its impact on relationships. Both women were diagnosed with cancer at a young age, faced their own mortality, and needed a strong team around them. What is refreshing is the language they use to describe what happens as time passes and needs continue. I listened to a podcast they did together called "You Are Not the Bad Thing" and nodded the entire way through. Here are some of their takeaways.

✓ *Recognize the damage caused*

Patients powering through treatment, especially if it continues for an extended time and takes its inevitable detours, can begin to feel like "too much," a burden dragging those we love down. It can fracture precious relationships over time.

When the goalpost keeps moving, there is a sense of *ongoingness*. Both women speak about the challenges of being two to three years out as the toughest. Whatever you're feeling in a given moment, there's a good chance someone else out there feels the same.

There can be a sense of gratitude to everyone who helped and yet also one of resentment. It's hard to live in that period "when people wanted to move on and I couldn't." It's not unusual to "narrow the circle" of those close to you to those who "get it."

✓ *Have the difficult conversations*

Listening to these very wise survivors reminds us that cancer affects everyone. And while it can build some relationships, the longer it goes on, the greater the toll it takes. There's only so much a person can take before reaching a breaking point. Be honest with yourself and others. Did someone let you down and was it just because they didn't have the capacity to help? Did others make huge sacrifices that perhaps you took for grant-ed? Was there anyone who needed you and you didn't have the strength to get to them? Did you have children who might have been struggling and didn't dare tell you? Whether you answered yes or no to any or all of these, remember it's okay. It's not too late. Talk to your people. Don't just sweep important conversations under the rug. Communication is supposed to be hard in families, let alone families managing illness. Be courageous. Speak up. Break the silence.

HIGHLIGHTS FROM BRENÉ BROWN

bestselling author, social scientist, and notable expert on vulnerability, empathy, shame, and courage

As one of my favorite storytellers and podcasters, Brené Brown's wisdom speaks to me and has helped me think through some of my darkest moments. She holds a PhD in social work and is a research professor at the University of Houston, where she's the Huffington Foundation Endowed Chair. Her 2010 TEDx talk, "The Power of Vul-nerability," is one of the five most viewed TED talks. When it comes to resetting your life, her insights offer a framework. Here are three pieces of advice from her that have resonated with me and can help you find clarity in this next phase of your life in survivorship.

Own your story:
   You've just been through a harrowing journey. As much as you want to ring the bell and run from it all, think about how you can use the experience to crystalize your new needs and wants in survivor-ship mode. Brené teaches "courage over comfort," but her definition of courage is not the typical one that's associated with bravery.

Such a definition "fails to recognize the inner strength and level of commitment required for us to actually speak honestly and openly about who we are and about our experiences—good and bad." Have the courage to speak openly about what you've just gone through even if it means exploring the darkness and it makes you feel vulnerable. According to Brené, "you have to walk through vulnerability to get to courage." And that courage will ultimately help you check your reset boxes.

Know the difference between shame and guilt:
  As you enter your survivorship and look back at the debris field of your cancer journey, you might feel ashamed of some of your behaviors in your time of crisis. You may feel like you treated a few people badly, overstepped boundaries, and failed to fully appreciate those who helped you through it. Rather than label those feelings as shame, try to reframe them around guilt. Brené's own research shows that there's a big difference between shame and guilt. Shame is "the intensely painful feeling or experience of believing that we are flawed and therefore unworthy of love and belonging—something we've experienced, done, or failed to do makes us unworthy of connection." Shame is neither helpful nor productive, and can actually be a source of destructive behavior. Guilt, on the other hand, "is adaptive and helpful—it's holding something we've done or failed to do up against our values and feeling psychological discomfort." Guilt is good. So as you reset and reengage, have compassion for yourself and be okay with the guilt. Use it to optimize your reset. It's a tool for transformation—for making smarter decisions, for sharpening your sense of meaning and purpose, and for deepening your most vital relationships.

Think of your relationships in terms of percentages:
  During a 2023 interview that quickly went viral, Brené broke the widely accepted rule that says marriage should be fifty-fifty. She

declared "marriage is never fifty-fifty," going on to explain that she and her partner routinely "quantify" where they are so they can each adjust accordingly. For example, when her partner comes home and says he's at 20 percent in terms of energy, patience, and kindness, she can either carry the balance of 80 percent to reach a combined 100 percent or they can "sit down at the table and figure out a plan of kindness toward each other." As you reset your relationships, especially those closest to you that you want to nourish and grow, think in terms of percentages. Relationships work best when you can carry someone else's 80 percent when necessary or they can carry your deficit. Some days, for whatever reason, you're only at a 10 and you have to hope your partner can "cover you" at a 90. If you are both at 10, that's when you want to chat.

Back to School

As he reached his senior year, David was participating in the end-of-summer baseball tournaments, his final step to getting recruited to college as an athlete. He had been injured during the junior year recruiting season—two stress fractures in his L2 vertebra—and was declared finished for the season. Crushed. No games, no playoffs. Nothing. As we drove him home from the doctor's office, tears cascaded down his face; later his bedroom door closed. My quiet knocks went unanswered. David had one more challenge he had to overcome. And these games were the last chance for the final few coaches still interested to see him. There'd be only a small window of opportunities for him to prove he was worthy of their team and school. He was officially down to the wire and out of runway.

Always good under pressure, David nailed it. Paul and I were both blown away by his unflappableness as he walked to the mound for the first time in months knowing that the next fifteen to twenty pitches would determine his direction. I was working at home when David came running up the stairs itching to share the good news.

"Coach Kinney just called. I'm in!"

I jumped from my desk, hugging him and screaming. The joy on his face was something I'd been waiting years to see. The injury, the recovery, the stress of being "on" when the right person was watching. It is the one dream David has had since he first hit the ball off the tee with his dad: playing baseball for as long as he can.

Nicole was now in her sophomore year in college. I was speeding up the Mass Pike to catch her before seeing her cheer at the big rivalry game. I would meet Paul later, as he'd be arriving late after watching David at a baseball tournament. By now I could drive the route to Boston blindfolded. Between the frequent visits to Dana-Farber and watching Nicole cheer at both football and basketball games, Paul and I had seen her relatively often. Freshman year had its growing pains but I was confident things would only get better as Nicole coasted more comfortably into sophomore year.

I was picturing trying to find her between the alumni tent and the football field, amidst the parades, Fan Day festivities, and endless tailgates, bracing for the inevitable tension in the air (literally) because Nicole strived for perfection in her routine. This was not about looking pretty and dancing casually on the sidelines. This was about physicality—nailing the basket tosses, tumbling passes, and doing three standing back tucks in a row. She demanded the best of herself and never wanted to let her team down. I was so happy to see her no matter how brief the visit.

As I came close to my destination, I was taking another call from a myeloma patient seeking my help. I'd been on the phone for the entire three-hour drive. While I had decided to step back from my role as CEO, I could never say no to patients. And as my commitment in the myeloma world continued to grow, it meant more calls from more patients who were struggling and relapsing. I always kept a list with their numbers so I could multitask while on the road; otherwise, there was no other way to get back to everyone. This particular patient had also been through a grueling transplant with a sibling but was facing relapse with no obvious shortcut to remission again. Could I find a solution for him? The intensity of the moment made me miss my exit. I didn't have any good news for him to lean on. Then, just as I hung up with a heavy heart, the phone rang again. It was Karen. We hadn't spoken in a week, an eternity for us.

"Are you with Katy?" I asked, knowing she was also on a visit to her daughter's college that weekend. She stopped me right away.

"Kathy, I've been trying to reach you. Where have you been? Why haven't you called me back?"

"Work has been crazy. I'm so busy. Sorry." (I'd later come to loathe the excuse "I'm so busy.") "I'm trying to get to—"

"I have breast cancer," she said quickly, her voice wavering as she cut me off from ranting further. I pulled over to the shoulder to catch myself. *WTF?*

Step 10

Recognize Your Caregivers

How Can You Take Care of Them?

Every health challenge, small and large, takes a toll on the patient, the family, and the extended support system. The roles of patient and caregiver are decidedly different and hard to understand until you've been both. As a patient, having empathy for your primary caregivers is important. They are volunteering out of the goodness of their hearts and they often take on a lot—more than expected or what they were formally trained for. Caregiving may be completely new to them; how they handle it depends on their experience to date and how they are related to you. Your spouse's approach, for example, might be completely different from your child's or your sister's or your closest friend's. You might not even have someone you feel comfortable asking to take the lead role in your care. Some patients who live largely independently may find themselves at a loss when they suddenly need to rely on others and don't have that individual already built into their lives. And it all walks a fine line. The caregiver-patient dynamic is just that—dynamic, ever-changing, and emotional.

On the one hand, caregivers may feel joy and pleasure in feeling needed, in knowing they are helping someone they care about deeply. On the other hand, however, there can be feelings of "no control"—of simply not understanding how to help, where to step in, and when. They can be fearful watching you struggle and praying they don't lose you. They might want you to fight more, or less. Often, they quietly carry too much of the burden, which creates hidden anger and resentment. They may even suffer their own health struggles as a result of the added responsibilities and stress. Caregivers can prioritize the patient at their own expense.

As patients, the best thing we can do is communicate our needs clearly, often, and thoroughly. And show gratitude. As caregivers, the best thing we can do is speak up, and articulate our own needs as precisely as possible, because as much as we want to help the patient in our lives, we have our own needs, too. It's okay—actually, it's critical—that you admit when you're reaching that maximal point of your own stress, your own worries, maybe your own health issues. Chances are that caregivers are rarely helping just one "patient." They are often juggling a few people in their day-to-day lives, such as their own family members including parents and children. Caregivers need care, too.

My Sister Has Breast Cancer

Those four words—"I have breast cancer"—that my sister blurted out to me on the drive to an otherwise festive event sunk my heart even further down following my call with the myeloma patient. I think my heart lurched forward, too, as if trying to reach out to her. Here was my best friend, my confidante, my *twin*, now in the suffering seat while raising three kids on her own. In a reversal of misfortune, she needed me now and I'd been "too busy to return a quick call." I did not see this coming, not even after all she had done for me and my salvation.

"Are you fucking kidding me?" I said, the guilt punching me in the gut. "I'm so sorry." My remorse was overpowering knowing that I'd been answering everyone else's calls except my sister's. I never dreamed she could be calling about having cancer. I instinctively shifted into navigator mode, firing away questions.

"How did you find out? What have they said? What stage? Is it early? Which hospital did you use?"

"They found it on a mammogram at the local hospital. I knew something was wrong as soon as they put me in a separate room."

While still pulled over to the side of the road, I searched for a scrap of paper in the crevices of my car, wondering why I was always driving and taking frantic notes.

"It's small—fourteen millimeters—and I'm just hoping it's early," Karen added. "I don't know what stage yet."

I pictured her mind racing from thought to thought as she scrambled to pull herself together for her daughter. Like me so many times over, Karen was now the one trying to be normal while her heart was cracking. I sensed her urgency and tangible fear like they were my own. It was a mirror and a window all at once.

"We've got this," I assured her. My words were a carbon copy of what she'd said to me years before. "Let me get to campus, send out a few emails and texts, and I will call you first thing tomorrow. I promise, it's going to be okay."

Karen officially became the patient and I was now the caregiver, researcher, coordinator, driver, calendar helper, standby surrogate mother, advocate, and beat-down-the-door-to-get-the-best-care crusader for Karen's right treatment. In an exacting, seesaw role reversal, she netted the knot in the stomach and I became saddled with the fear of losing her, the struggle of watching her suffer, and the need to make sure her children knew we'd get through this. We'd take the worry away whenever and wherever we could. It's just part of being a mom. And for Karen, even harder, now a single mom.

As I sat in the parking lot with this news that reshuffled my priorities, I fired off emails to the myeloma leaders at each of the New York centers asking them to connect me to their breast cancer teams. The next morning, I followed my playbook. I googled "just diagnosed with early-stage breast cancer" and clicked immediately on the American Cancer Society site followed by BreastCancer.org. I wrote furious notes in my notebook marked "Karen's breast cancer" and drafted all my questions in the right-hand margin so I could come back to them—checking them off along the way. The only words that I could start with based on my conversation with Karen were "invasive ductal carcinoma, or IDC." She was still waiting for the lab results from the needle biopsy done at her local hospital. And while the sites explained each word of I-D-C, it was hard to understand the next steps and where to take them. My playbook drew a blank to fill.

I explained to Karen that our next step was to find the best doctor. We scheduled appointments at Memorial Sloan Kettering (MSK), Weil Cornell, and Mt. Sinai. Meanwhile, Karen reached out to friends she thought could be helpful. She wanted to wait and see which doctor she liked and trusted, which center gave her a good feeling, and who seemed best at her specific breast cancer.

Our urgency picked up a few days later. Karen and I had been invited to a big American Cancer Society fundraiser honoring Deborah Norville, who had been so supportive of us at the MMRF. I was seated at the table with Deborah chatting away when Karen walked in with a forced smile and hasty hug. I saw something in her eyes and mouthed "Are you okay?" across the table.

"I'm Stage III," she mouthed back, her eyes welling up. And just like that neither of us could eat let alone manage to smile and get through the festivities of the lunch. Normalcy had been eviscerated. There was no plastering over the panic. As the lunch ended, we raced toward the lobby and Karen exploded in front of me, her whole body shaking.

"I just went from a little something to a full-on nightmare," she said. "They called me while I was in the car with Tyler and told me they found the cancer in eight lymph nodes. I'm so screwed." The tears streamed down her face as she continued. "How the hell am I going to handle this? Tyler should be focusing on school, not taking care of me. How do I tell JJ and Katy when they are off at college? I can't just call them."

I let her purge all the concerns and unknowns that had erupted at the top of her mind. Karen would have to act fast and figure out health insurance needs she lacked. "What about my job?" she went on. "The insurance? I don't have anyone to help me."

"Yes, you do," I explained calmly. "I'm here. I'm not going to leave you. We've got this—it's what I do. Let's start with the right doctor."

Based on our combined research, Dr. Larry Norton at MSK became one of our targets. I knew Dr. Norton from cancer conferences and had sat on a few good panels with him. He'd gained an illustrious reputation in the breast cancer field and cared deeply about his patients. As we headed into his office, he announced that he had limited time because he had a black-tie fundraiser that night. My mind went to the reality: *As soon as doctors reach the pinnacle in their field, they get dragged into the fundraising circuit and taken out of the clinic.* Norton, however, did not disappoint. He had his computer up and ready. He had read Karen's entire history and laid out the options for her as clearly as possible: lumpectomy or mastectomy, followed by some combination of chemo, radiation, and hormone therapy with follow-up treatments that would vary depending on the results. Karen picked the lumpectomy route, grounding her decision with the best information she had at that moment and based on where she was in her life. A new job was about to begin in weeks, making the time for recovery from major surgery impractical. What helped in the decision-making process was knowing that MSK had a satellite center that was a spectacular fifteen short minutes from her home—a true satellite center. Better still, Norton would be "on call" whenever she needed him.

The Cancer Twins and the Sibling Switch

Once team and treatment decisions were made, the actual hand-holding part of caregiving began. I gave my bag of beautiful scarves—a cornucopia of spectacular florals and artful geometrics—matching every sweater I owned to Karen. I bought her the soft warm blanket I knew she needed to take with her on appointments to buffer against any chill. As I watched my best friend and soulmate stay as strong as possible, I caught every emotion—every beat to beating this thing, from the waiting game for results and the lousy side effects from the drugs, to the chronic fear of dying, to the unavoidable anxiety around the burden she felt her illness placed on others.

But at the same time, I also was acutely aware that every person's journey is their own. I couldn't possibly know what was really going on in her head. She'd just left the starting line, whereas I was in complete remission. She was a single mom in a new job trying to make a name for herself all over again whereas I had a devoted, working husband. She had two children in college and she didn't want them to worry while they were away, nor did she want to burden Tyler with the ups and downs of the lengthy treatments. And knowing how to help, and when to help, was not always easy.

Karen kept a coterie of dear friends and even had a boyfriend who wanted to make sure she was okay. Tyler was thankfully home every day and immediately stepped into the role of caregiver while JJ and Katy were in constant contact. I gave a lot of thought to how I could best serve her on the "roster" of caregivers without stepping on anyone's toes. Reflecting back on my own experience through the transplant, I recalled how I loved Karen alternating with Paul. They worked so well together as a team, each with their own style of caregiving and time for themselves in their rotation. And it gave each of them a break and time to get back home to work and the kids. I tried to do the same, alternating visits with Karen's other people while I filled in the caregiving blanks.

She received her chemo at the local MSK hospital. We sat together watching TV and sent smiling selfies to the kids and cousins to let them know she was doing okay. And we spent hours talking about the kids, her fears, how messed up it was that the two of us were the unlucky twins. The cancer twins.

Karen soldiered through the treatments as the holidays approached and the older kids came home. It was another Christmas with the cancer cloud hovering above us. Her hair began to fall out, her skin dried up, and she was nauseated often and relentlessly, and that only added to the exhaustion. Her kids came up with an idea: take Mom to get her head shaved. We made an event of it and went together into New York City. I held her hand while the remaining strands fell to the floor. Karen smiled and cried at the same time and I watched her children trying to be brave when they had already watched the toll these treatments took on me when I was in treatment. We then found the perfect wig and headed out to admire the Rockefeller Center Christmas tree a block away. We took photos as if everything was normal.

But when I sent the photos to Nicole and David, I was surprised by their silence. No quick response, which was unlike them. I called Nicole.

"Mom," Nicole explained. "You're identical twins. You brought us right back to our own Christmas PTSD when you were doing your transplant. We are the ones living with wondering if you both might die."

I was stumped, speechless. She was right. How could I have been so blind? I could barely deliver a response other than to agree, and that I understood where she was coming from. I had struggled to grasp what Nicole had been through, or what she was currently going through. She and David were caregivers, too. But I was only beginning to understand what it was like to stand in their shoes.

The Tables Have Turned

Let's face it, you can't know what it's like to be a patient until you become one. But neither can you know what it's like to be a primary caregiver until you become that, too. Neither role is easy. They both have their challenges and rewards. The patient-caregiver relationship is incredibly personal. And everyone's experience is different.

My myeloma journey was long thanks to my smoldering state. My primary caregivers, especially Paul and Karen, rode it with me all the way through. Paul and I had to work together to achieve both the needs and the wants we'd established back at the beginning of my cancer journey. He also always made himself available for the endless doctor appointments, driving me where I needed to go, taking notes, picking up meds. Karen was my sounding board every time tests came back unusual. She was my side-by-side guinea pig going through the tests and my provider of a new immune system. When transplant time came around, they were both in fifth gear giving up anything and everything else around them, living at the hospital, driving back and forth from Boston to Connecticut, worrying about all five cousins together. And my steadfast group of friends, *the eight,* were always there to make me smile, bring me food, and go for walks.

Being a caregiver for my sister was a gift—finally, some actual payback for all she'd done for me. It was hard for Karen to let anyone in. Probably because she knew how much my needs drained her, she didn't want to do the same to me. But as a single mom, trying to raise three children and pay multiple college tuitions, she had a lot on her plate. She needed me most for her research, for finding the doctors when we needed to chase them down with questions, and joining her on some of the tougher treatment appointments. If I came to realize anything, it was how important it is for the patient to constantly communicate what they need. With as much advance notice as they can. And delegate. It's so hard to delegate clearly. Everyone wants to help but it's hard to react to surprises in a busy world.

In the writing of this book, Nicole shared some of her choicest advice in being a caregiver: "There's a difference between caregiving and sacrificing. You must do things that bring you joy when you're a caregiver or you'll burn out and resent the situation you're in. With caregiving, you have to take away the guilt of taking care of yourself. Only then can you be there for the person who is relying on you."

Now here are the WTDs for taking care of your caregivers.

STEP 10: RECOGNIZE YOUR CAREGIVERS

WTDs

Know Your Caregiving Needs

X You need a knowledge partner

X You need a logistics partner

X You need an emotional support partner

Know and Respect Your Caregivers' Needs

X Know your primary caregiver's wants and needs

X Expand your team to share the burden

X Communicate clearly and often

X Have empathy

X Show appreciation

Get Outside Support

X Online support

X Palliative care resources

X Respite care

X Hospice care

X Family and Medical Leave Act

WTD 1: Know Your Caregiving Needs

We've talked a lot about the importance of your personal support team. But equally important is understanding and communicating your specific caregiving needs. What you will need will typically fall into specific categories:

✓ *You need a knowledge partner*

Having someone who can help research your disease and serve as a sounding board can help you think about your medical decisions more clearly. You may have a family member, child, or friend who is savvy on a computer and can help you stay on top of your disease, treatments, and new trials that might emerge. You're looking for someone who is not scared of the science lingo and willing to sort through it to answer questions you might have. This individual can also be very helpful on those doctor visits where you have to make an important decision. You may want to give them access to your medical records. To do so, you will need them to sign a specific form at the doctor's office.

✓ *You need a logistics partner*

Just dealing with basic logistics while dealing with cancer can be overwhelming. Having someone to help makes a huge difference.

→ **Medical errands**: While you may feel well enough to drive yourself or use public transportation, there will be days when you don't. You need to know who can help. Who can drive you to the doctor's office, to the hospital? Who can pick up your prescriptions for you?

→ **Coverage battles**: Battling it out with the insurance companies and Medicare/Medicaid can be exhausting. Can one person help take this on for you? Can you get one person on the payor side to serve as your case manager?

→ **Family needs**: While you're battling your own disease, you might also be taking care of your parents, your partner, or young children. Depending on where your life is, you need people to step in and support them while you can't. You can't do it all so having a support plan here becomes critical.

✓ *You need an emotional support partner*

Know who you can talk to. You're looking for that person who understands you, relieves the stress, and even makes you smile. These are the people you turn to when you're having a tough day or a good day.

WTD 2: Know and Respect Your Caregivers' Needs

According to a study by the NCI, there were 2.8 million cancer care-givers in the US as of 2015. That number is only growing. The study showed that cancer caregivers are typically unpaid family members or friends (as opposed to nurses) and carry a heavy burden, giving 32.9 hours each week to caregiving, communicating with healthcare professionals on behalf of the patient (62 percent), and helping in making end-of-life decisions (40 percent).

Laurel Northhouse, a nurse scientist at the University of Michigan School of Nursing who was not involved in the study but who offered a comment for the NCI's media, wrote: "The intensity of the cancer caregiver experience can lead to emotional distress among caregivers, which can, in turn, affect the patient's well-being." While more research emerges on this important topic, it underscores how important it is to understand and respect your caregivers' needs. Here are ways you can reduce stress on your caregivers:

✓ *Know your primary caregiver's wants and needs*

You may select one primary caregiver or maybe two. Often, this is a family member living with you or nearby. While it's good to have a specific lead for caregiving, it can also increase the burden on this one person. At a minimum, know their ability to help. How will they support you while still going to work or helping with other familial duties? What are their limitations? How can they let you know when they, too, are getting tired and run-down?

✓ *Expand your team to share the burden*

To reduce the burden on your primary caregiver, try to recruit others for support. If you have other family members or friends who can step in on certain days off or weekends, take them up on that. Schedule appointments on those weekdays to relieve your primary caregiver. Allow them to come over on specific days to help you or just visit while your caregiver gets freed up. Allow them to set a simple schedule to help with meals, go on walks, take care of your pets. People want to help. Let them.

✓ *Communicate clearly and often*

Once you know how your caregiving team likes to communicate, be sure to update them with changes consistently and let them know how your journey's detours are impacting the schedule. Your ability to get ahead and allow them to adjust their own schedules goes a long way.

✓ *Have empathy*

Be aware that the caregiver burden can increase with certain factors. Older caregivers may have health issues of their own, fatigue faster, and have a higher likelihood of having or developing depression. Middle-aged caregivers worry about missing work and may need to take a leave of absence they can't afford. Younger caregivers are juggling work and family and are most likely going to be sacrificing a good chunk of their social lives. They need to know you understand *their* needs as much as you need them to understand *your* needs.

✓ *Show appreciation*

Say thank you in whatever way is authentic for you. It might be a hug, a personal note, or just a text. Do it all along the way. Don't wait or assume they know how much their support means to you. Show them.

WTD 3: Get Outside Support

Caregivers need caregiving, too. There are multiple services that can help, either by offering your caregiver much-needed counseling and support or giving them relief by providing additional support care for you. Here are a few options for caregiver support:

✓ *Online support*

There are many online resources for cancer caregivers. Here are some excellent options:

→ **Cancer Survivors Network** (csn.cancer.org): Sponsored by the American Cancer Society, this online community of people whose lives have been touched by cancer offers caregivers a place to go for advice but also to feel less alone.

→ **CancerCare** (cancercare.org): free caregiver support services, including counseling, support groups, and educational resources for people affected by cancer

→ **Cancer Support Community** (cancersupportcommunity.org): free support services, including counseling, support groups, and educational resources including information on coping strategies and practical advice

→ **Caregiver Action Network** (caregiveraction.org): education and support, including caregiver tip sheets, educational webinars, and a directory of support groups

→ **Family Caregiver Alliance** (caregiver.org): resources including legal and financial issues, and caregiver health and wellness

→ **National Cancer Institute** (cancer.gov): The "Resources for Caregivers" section has information on caregiving roles and responsibilities, managing side effects, and coping with end-of-life issues.

✓ *Palliative care resources*

Palliative care, also called comfort care, can begin as soon as the person is diagnosed with a terminal illness. It provides an extra layer of support and focuses on quality of life, helping with symptoms and supporting the family as they make treatment decisions. Palliative care can be provided at the hospital or at home and can be covered by insurance, Medicare, and Medicaid.

To learn more, visit the National Hospice and Palliative Care website.

✓ *Respite care*

ACS also recommends seeking out respite care that might be available in your community. Respite care is "short-term temporary relief for those who are caring for family members who might otherwise need professional care." Respite care workers can help with basic patient needs and, importantly, offer companionship while the caregiver takes some time for themselves.

✓ Hospice care

Hospice or end-of-life care provides physical, psychosocial, and spiritual care for the person dying and for the family. It often begins when the patient has less than six months to live.

✓ Family and Medical Leave Act

You may want to investigate the Family and Medical Leave Act (FMLA) program if you work at a large corporation where it is more likely to be available. FMLA guarantees twelve weeks off per year to take care of a seriously ill spouse, parent, or child.

IN CONVERSATION WITH PATRICIA GOLDSMITH

Chief Executive Officer of CancerCare.org

For more than thirty years, Patricia Goldsmith has been a staunch advocate for patients and the people who support them through a cancer journey. As a cancer survivor herself, she knows that getting through a diagnosis is a team effort. I was thrilled to have her input on some of the most important members of the team: your caregivers.

Q. What do patients overlook in choosing their personal caregiving team?

A.   Most patients have their go-to person for the journey, typically a spouse or best friend. And we tend to take these people for granted when we need their help through an illness. While it's natural to depend largely on people you know and love, it's important that you divvy up the weight of your cancer journey so no single person feels too overwhelmed. They are also people who have needs and value their time. You need to support them just as they support you.

Q.   How does your organization help caregivers?

A.   Our strength is providing free access to our more than forty trained oncology social workers with master's degrees who can truly help not only patients but their caregivers throughout the entire cancer experience. In fact, we have a lot of resources, information, and support services designed specifically for caregivers and loved ones. They can also join support groups led by our professionals, as well as access additional information through teleconferences, video conferences, workshops, and brochures. Overcoming cancer is a lot more than the treatment itself for the patient. The journey affects everyone around them who is helping out. Caregivers are often "secondary patients"— the people who juggle a lot of challenges and silent stress in their devotion to the job. They need support and guidance, too. We actually have an online tool they can use to help track, monitor, and manage their sources of strain and find ways to improve their well-being. Caregivers with the right support will be better caregivers but also be better themselves.

Q.   In addition to relying on friends and family for your primary caregiving, who else should patients think about to help round out their care?

A.   Just as you have a multidisciplinary medical team helping you get through treatment, you want the same on the personal side, including resources beyond your inner, built-in circle. In other words, reach out to professional support services so you're not overburdening your loved ones. Lean on social workers, the nursing staff, navigators, and support communities for cancer patients. Many disease-specific foundations will offer services that can help take some of the load off others. Think about depending on these free services for some rides to treatment, pharmacy deliveries, and other logistics. If you're a person of faith, think about how your clergy and members of your church or faith community can support you. You'd be surprised by who will show up to offer to help, and you may even find new lifelong friends through this process. Give people specific tasks that revolve around their expertise, and don't forget to show appreciation. Say thank you and find ways to give back.

※

A Bouquet of Roses and the Next Calls

Karen's final treatment was radiation. On her last ring-the-bell day, I got up early, grabbed the big bouquet of pink roses I'd bought the night before, and raced to the center. When she finally came out and saw me there, she sobbed. I hadn't told her I was coming, or that I even knew it was her last treatment. But I had written it down. I wasn't going to miss it. The gesture was less about celebrating her last treatment day (for now) and more about showing her that I'd always be there. She has a photo of us from that day that sits on her bookshelf because it reminds her not of her cancer, but of how much my being there meant to her.

No sooner did Karen get through her journey than I received a call from my mom. She had been battling melanoma for years, being seen every six months by her dermatologist for lots of cutting and freezing of spots on her face, scalp, and arms. This time, the issue was more serious. The melanoma was in her eye and could easily travel the optic nerve to the brain. They wanted her to have surgery immediately. Once again, I started searching for the right center, the right doctors. We needed a good academic hospital near her in Pennsylvania. Thankfully, I found an entire team of experts at the

University of Pennsylvania who could handle the surgery and save her vision. Who knew there was an oculoplastic surgeon who did just this? I am still blown away by the caliber of their work. I still have the selfie on my phone that we took together in our ugly blue surgical caps as we waited to meet the doctors one last time before she headed into the OR. We were smiling big because she wanted me to send it to the five cousins telling them she was just fine and going to see them soon. And once again, I was grateful that while I was in charge of finding the best medical care, Karen and Paul were with me on those Philadelphia overnights making sure she was okay.

And then came the next call. This time it was the White House. After years of working with various government channels, including the National Cancer Advisory Board under President George Bush, it was not unusual for me to speak with someone calling from the administration. But this time the call was about Obama's newly formed Precision Medicine Initiative (PMI). Obama was launching a bold new research effort to revolutionize how we treat disease. If they wanted me involved, I could not say no. The MMRF had become the model of how precision medicine could change the course of a single cancer. If I could have the same impact across all cancers, let alone all diseases, count me in. Between my father's kidney cancer, my mom's melanoma, Karen's breast cancer, and my myeloma, keeping our family safe was taking on new meaning.

Step 11

Never Miss a Screening

What Do I Watch Out for Now?

As you move through your diagnosis and the necessary treatments, understand that your body may never be quite the same. It may have affected your immune system, your heart or kidney function, even your cognition and memory. Dealing with cancer and its barrage of tough treatments might make you prone to secondary cancers. These are new cancers that emerge that are different from the original cancer. This could be due to overlapping risk factors (for example, breast and ovarian cancer in particular share multiple risk factors) or the treatment for the first cancer having made you vulnerable for other emerging cancers. Radiation, for instance, to one body part can disrupt other tissues in the same area and raise the risk of developing a new cancer there or nearby. A commonly cited example is radiation therapy to the chest for Hodgkin's lymphoma or lung cancer that leads to breast cancer years later. Chemotherapy is also known to raise the risk for blood cancers, more so than radiation. These are yet more reasons why, following treatment, you'll never be the same again. The good news is there's still life on the other side.

While you are no longer living in doctor's offices, it is important to know the screenings you should be having, especially based on your new risk profile. I say "new risk profile" because your body is now a different "new" specimen. But even if you haven't had cancer, it's important to know what screenings you should be having at every age. Remember, every time you are screened for cancer, be it a blood test, scan, or specific screening related to your specific family history or genetic risk, you're seizing an opportunity. And if you miss such an opportunity, a disease could go unnoticed until symptoms surface. Often, by that time, it may be too late. Surprisingly, not everyone agrees on the age and frequency of screening efforts like mammograms, PSA tests, or colonoscopies. Which is why it's important to work with an internist or primary care physician (PCP) who knows your entire medical history (more on that in Step 12), as well as a specialist in your specific area of high risk. You don't want to miss those opportunities to stop a disease in its tracks early. Although it's not fun to go through some of these screenings, some of which can be unpleasant or require preparation and time, you don't want to have to deal with the alternative—illness and/or premature death. The more you know, the more you stand to gain.

The Precision Medicine Initiative

When President Obama announced the Precision Medicine Initiative (PMI) in his State of the Union address at the start of 2015, the excitement was palpable. The mission was clear: "To enable a new era of medicine through research, technology, and policies that empower patients, researchers, and providers to work together toward development of individualized care." His commitment and the promise of funding made the effort more exciting. The goal was to find ways the government could accelerate precision medicine by building a national registry where the data could finally be shared. I was recommended for the steering committee because it was clear the MMRF's precision medicine approach to drug development was playing a critical role in saving patients' lives and driving us closer to a cure.

The meetings for PMI brought together the highest caliber of guests to share their insights. It was the who's who in oncology. While many of the meetings were held at the White House, others were run at centers doing great work in the field—centers that would become important contributors to the program. The timelines were tight, so we were expected to jump on planes and get to the next assignment at the drop of a hat. During one of the meetings held at Vanderbilt University in Nashville, we had moved through the morning sessions and were breaking for lunch when I caught sight of one of my old myeloma friends, Dr. Keith Stewart, across the room. A well-respected heme-onc clinician and researcher in the myeloma space, Stewart had a special interest in using genomics to customize care to a patient's genetic makeup. It was not surprising that he'd been promoted to direct the Precision Medicine Institute at the Mayo Clinic.

When he saw me, he came over to say hello. I'd long admired and thought the world of this dedicated doctor whose work has been published in hundreds of scientific papers. He was one of the most collaborative doctors I'd worked with in myeloma and a strong reason for our success at the MMRF. He had both an MD and an MBA, allowing him to understand the unique incentives and business models we strived to build at the foundation. He'd made his footprints throughout his training in Glasgow, Kingston, Toronto, and Boston, and had earned international respect in many healthcare leadership roles.

"Let's catch up on the steps outside while we eat," Stewart said, his signature Scottish brogue exuding pure gentleness. As we moved outside, he asked how my family was doing. He was one of the most empathetic doctors I knew.

"All is good," I said. "The kids are doing well with college and sports, and the MMRF keeps me busy." Then I told him about Karen. "My sister was diagnosed with breast cancer. Stage III."

"I'm so sorry to hear this. What is she doing for treatment?"

"She had a lumpectomy followed by chemo and radiation and

now the aromatase inhibitors." He nodded along as I spoke. As a clinician and researcher, his mind went exactly where mine should have gone months and months ago.

"What about you?" he asked.

I looked at him inquisitively.

He went on, "You realize that if your identical twin has breast cancer, you should be getting screened yourself. You are officially high risk. You should at least be seeing a breast surgeon in addition to your regular OBGYN, someone who knows exactly what they're looking for."

"I honestly hadn't even thought about it," I replied, feeling ridiculously naïve and ignorant. How does someone run a research foundation and not think this through? I did tell him that Karen had been tested for the BRCA gene and did not carry it. From that small piece of information, I felt I was safe.

"Remember our grandfather on our mom's side had myeloma," I continued. "Our grandmother on our father's side had breast cancer. I have asked Ken Anderson and Larry Norton if there is interest in learning more here but it's hard to make connections and it's not their area of interest."

He then offered to do full genomic sequencing on both Karen and me, our mother, and Nicole and David. It became a fascinating effort that unveiled new scientific findings about our shared DNA, but also highlighted the psychosocial challenges of learning information that you might not want to know. For Stewart, he was curious about why identical twins developed two different types of cancer. For me, I was intent on gathering as many clues about my family as possible to help predict future outcomes and to be prepared. But for my family members, not everyone was on board. My children opted out of the sequencing for the time being. Young and healthy, they'd take their time before learning about their genetic blueprint.

With Dr. Stewart's thoughts in my head that afternoon, I went through the list of breast surgeons I had seen with Karen, eventually landing with Dr. Elisa Port at Mt. Sinai in New York, who directs the Dubin Breast Center. I gravitated toward her direct approach and attitude. And I could get to her office without traffic in ninety minutes, which was much faster than the three-hour drive to Boston. After a physical and detailed history, Port gave her perspective.

"Of course, having an identical twin with breast cancer in her fifties is a risk. But your greatest risk is actually the radiation you had to your ribs years ago for your myeloma. Back then we didn't know how much protection to provide to the surrounding tissue."

"This is the first I'm hearing this." Yet another *WTF!*

"You also have dense breasts, which adds a bit of challenge, too."

I asked about other risks I had read about online. "And what about my doing IVF, all those hormones? Or the risk of my grandmother having the disease?" I asked.

"The risk of IVF remains unproven," she explained, "and your grandmother got breast cancer in old age, so we're really not sure how much risk they add."

Her summary was clear and consistent, and we decided to start with a mammogram first and then do an MRI in six months. This would be the strategy going forward as I began to incorporate the breast cancer screenings along with my myeloma blood tests. I tried scheduling my mammogram every January and my MRI every July to make it easier. That was also when I did my screenings for melanoma—another issue that was prone to secondary cancers.

When the first round of scans came back clean, I felt some relief, but there soon came a time when the MRI caught something suspicious. Dr. Port's call came in while I was busy helping Nicole pack for her move to Uganda. Yes, Uganda. After college, she was desperate to take a break from Boston and really get away. She wanted to do something daring. She applied to the Global Healthcare Initiative and earned a fellowship in maternal health. She was excited and petrified at the same time. This was not the time to talk about another cancer.

Once Paul and I got her off to the program, I went in for the needle biopsy. I remember being asked to lie face-down on the MRI table with the hopes that my breasts would fall through for the best view of what was going on. Nothing fell through. I had nothing to fall through. The nurses and doctors struggled to get the biopsy done but it was challenging and painful with the awkward angles; the results were not great. It was then that Port felt I would need to do surgical biopsies for my care. Surgical biopsies are more challenging because you are back in the hospital and under anesthesia. There is also some recovery time, and to be approved, you need an EKG and blood testing from your primary care doctor. Fortunately, for me, I had just switched to a new internist who had started at our local Stamford Hospital. My friend Tiffany had raved about Dr. Deena Ebright and a few of us started seeing her. Nicole and David as well.

As I headed into Dr. Ebright's office to discuss what was happening with my breast cancer screenings, she shared with me that she carried the BRCA gene and underwent a double mastectomy years prior. She encouraged me to continue taking the screening seriously and agreed the radiation to my ribs was something to consider. She asked to make sure all information from Mt. Sinai came her way. Ebright became my calm in the storm during any and all medical issues. Her demeanor and "no judgment" approach was a gift for any patient. And her office was well run, able to adjust to some of the fire drills of needing things like EKGs quickly.

I breathed a sigh of relief when that first biopsy came back as benign. But I was beginning to see this was not necessarily going to be a simple January/July visit. I basically alternated heading to Boston one month and New York another. And having learned that there can be false positives with the MRI (as many as 97 for every 1,000 cases), I needed to stay calm and quiet until all the tests were complete. I'd tell the kids that I was headed to either city for a "routine test," which was true. The older Nicole and David got the more

I realized lying is unacceptable, but waiting to share information at the right time is critical. It's best to share when you have a plan in front of you.

Know What to Screen For and When

The best way to cure cancer is to find it early. The best way to find it early is to get screened. And yet, people consistently miss their annual physicals and their screenings. My myeloma was found in a serendipitous way. Here I was trying to get approval from my internist to visit a fertility doctor or endocrinologist. And my internist had recently diagnosed another young female patient like me. When he saw my elevated protein and anemia, he knew to do more testing. It was incredibly fortunate, especially knowing that myeloma skews male, older, and African American. Today, primary care doctors are much more in tune with myeloma. They are consistently catching it much earlier.

My meeting with Keith Stewart was somewhat serendipitous, too. His advice may have helped save my life. Knowing I was high risk and should be seen by a high-risk breast-cancer team allowed me to get screened properly and ensured the insurance company covered my testing. Those screenings would ultimately detect my breast cancer in the earliest stages where curing it was an option. My primary care doctor did her best to remind me to get the visits done—to be vigilant in all my screenings in fact, from mammography to dermatology to colonoscopy. Whether you are being vigilant about finding a common cancer in your family early or looking for a secondary cancer, never miss a screening. Know every guideline and recommendation and work with your doctors to determine the right screenings for you. Here are WTDs for developing your screening plan.

STEP 11: NEVER MISS A SCREENING

WTDs

Know Your Risk

X Family history

X Personal history

X Medical history

Know the Basic Tests and Timing

X Breast cancer

X Cervical cancer

X Colorectal cancer

X Lung cancer

X Prostate cancer

X Skin cancer

Get the Right Screenings

X Make a screening plan with your doctor

X Schedule screenings in advance

X Use reminder services

X Take advantage of community screening events

WTD 1: Know Your Risk

Getting the right screening starts with knowing what to screen for. Here's how to better understand what you're at risk for:

✓ *Family history*

One of the most powerful ways to know your risk factors for diseases is by taking a good old-fashioned history of your family's health issues. See if you can trace your family tree back at least one generation of relatives to identify important health challenges that could be part of your makeup. Your family has genes in common. This means you might see trends in heart disease or cancer. You also have some behaviors in common and you might have lived in the same area. Has your mother or sister had breast cancer? Did your dad or brother get colon cancer before the age of fifty? This information can help direct your doctors in your care.

✓ *Personal history*

When you fill out the medical forms at the doctor's office, include every serious concern or disease you've had historically. You want to share any surgeries you've had, including how you reacted to anesthesia. You want to share any drug reactions or allergies you are aware of. It's important to include past concerns like viruses, stomach issues, and/or things like precancerous or cancer diagnoses. Make sure you answer questions about alcohol, drugs, diet, and sleep honestly. The more honest you are, the more the doctor can help you.

✓ *Medical history*

Your medical history combines your personal history and your family history. It may be kept by your primary care doctor or be part of your electronic health record (EHR). If you're unsure about this, you should review what your doctor has and make sure it's complete and updated. It should include all your past illnesses, medical procedures, family medical history, and current health status as well as any medications, allergies, and relevant personal lifestyle habits.

WTD 2: Know the Basic Tests and Timing

The Centers for Disease Control and Prevention (CDC) supports broad screening for breast, cervical, colorectal, and lung cancer as recommended by the US Preventive Services Task Force (USPSTF), a volunteer group of highly qualified physician advisors. Still, you can go to other websites or speak with your doctor and they might have different recommendations. Much depends on your medical history. Knowing what's right for you given ever-changing recommendations that can get confusing means having the conversation with your doctor in light of your history and personal risk factors. Here is a brief guide to basic screenings everyone should follow:

✓ *Breast cancer screening*

Mammography is an X-ray of the breast and is the most common form of screening. There are varying recommendations but the USPSTF states "women 50–74 years of age with an average risk of breast cancer, should get a mammogram every 2 years. Women 40–49 years of age should talk with their doctor." They also recommend taking an MRI for women at higher risk of breast cancer. If you are considered high risk, it's recommended you alternate mammogram with MRI typically every six months. And if you have what's called dense breasts, which can make traditional mammography less reliable because potential cancer can be more challenging to spot, you may have to undergo additional screenings such as whole breast ultrasound. A breast ultrasound in addition to mammography can improve detection of cancer. According to Dr. Elisa Port of the Dubin Cancer Center, mammograms can find 85 to 90 percent of cancers. It's not 100 percent but "no test is perfect"; if you're a high-risk patient, you need more screenings.

✓ *Cervical cancer screening*

The USPSTF also recommends getting your first Pap test at age 21, followed by a Pap test every three years. They recommend cervical screening for ages 30–65 years using one of the following approaches:

→ HPV test every five years
→ HPV/Pap co-test every five years
→ Pap test every three years

Updated guidelines from the ACS recommend screening starting at age 25 with an HPV test and then having HPV testing every 5 years through age 65. However, testing with an HPV/Pap co-test every 5 years or with a Pap test every 3 years is still acceptable.

✓ *Colorectal cancer screening*

The USPSTF notes that adults from ages 45 to 75 should be tested for colorectal cancer. This shift to starting at 45 years is a relatively new one, owing to an increase in colorectal cancer diagnoses among younger individuals for reasons scientists are still studying. The USPSTF also states that the decision to be screened after age 75 should be discussed with your doctor. There are a number of colorectal screening approaches, from traditional colonoscopies to at-home test kits for low-risk people. Colonoscopies remain the gold standard. They involve a flexible, lighted tube that checks for polyps or cancer in the colon and rectum. The recommended frequency varies so be sure to check with your doctor. When any less invasive tests show a positive test, you'll have to undergo a colonoscopy to confirm potential problems. The benefit to a colonoscopy over these other tests is that if polyps are found, they often can be removed on the spot.

✓ *Lung cancer screening*

The USPSTF recommends yearly lung cancer screening of low-dose computed tomography (LDCT) for people who are heavy smokers, who smoke now, or have quit in the past fifteen years and are between 50 and 80 years of age.

✓ *Prostate cancer screening*

Many men will get a PSA (prostate specific antigen) test to help screen for prostate cancer. The higher the PSA level in the blood, the more likely the patient has prostate cancer. Still, the PSA can vary based on age, race, an enlarged prostate, medications, and/or infection. It's important to do the screening and work with your doctor to analyze the results. If concern exists, your doctor will likely recommend a biopsy.

✓ *Skin cancer screening*

The American Academy of Dermatology recommends that adults undergo a full-body skin examination at least once a year to screen for skin cancer. It's also important to perform regular self-examinations of your skin at home. This involves checking your skin regularly for any new or changing spots, including moles, birthmarks, or freckles. If you have a history of skin cancer or other risk factors, such as fair skin, a history of sunburns, or a family history of skin cancer, your healthcare provider may recommend more frequent skin cancer screenings.

WTD 3: Get the Right Screenings

Yes, life gets busy. But catching cancer early is the easiest way to deal with it. Pick a day, week, or month, that you want to do all your screenings. Keep to this program every time and don't come up with excuses. The overall survival rates change dramatically from Stage I to Stage II or III. In early disease the cancer is often localized and easier to remove, while in later-stage disease the cancer may have spread to other parts of the body and is more difficult to treat. There is no question: Early screenings save lives. Just do them. Here are some tips to help ensure you never miss a cancer screening:

✓ **Make a screening plan with your doctor**

Talk to your primary care doctor about your personal risk factors and recommended screening schedule for different types of cancer. If you have a higher risk for a specific kind of cancer, you should also ask to consult a specialist.

✓ **Schedule screenings well in advance**

It's not always easy to get appointments. Schedule your cancer screenings months in advance, and make sure to mark them on your calendar or set reminders on your phone.

✓ **Use reminder services**

Many healthcare providers and screening centers offer reminder services, such as automated phone calls or text messages, to help you remember when it's time for your next screening.

✓ **Take advantage of community screening events**

Many communities offer free or low-cost cancer screening events, such as mammograms or skin cancer screenings. Check with your local health department or cancer center to see if there are any upcoming events in your area.

IN CONVERSATION WITH FOLASADE (FOLA) MAY

Director of the Melvin & Bren Simon Gastroenterology Quality Improvement Program in the UCLA Vatche and Tamar Manoukian Division of Digestive Diseases

Fola May, MD, PhD, MPhil, is a pioneering gastroenterologist who wears many hats as a physician, researcher, and quality improvement (QI) director. Digestive health and cancer prevention are her focus, as well as addressing health disparities. She has served as an expert in several media and policy settings, from mainstream media to the President's Cancer Panel on colorectal cancer, and the White House Cancer Moonshot. She knows a thing or two about cancer screenings because she happens to perform one of the most intimidating types that cause people to hit the delay button. It's why I wanted to talk to her and gain some insights.

Q.   People avoid or put off cancer screenings. As a gastroenterologist, you encourage people to get a colonoscopy for colorectal cancer screening when they are due for one. How do you motivate people to schedule them?

A.   No one wants to talk about it: a procedure through your anus. Talking about anything that has to do with that area of your body is taboo, especially in communities of color like mine. (In fact, Black individuals are more likely to develop and die from colorectal cancer than White individuals, largely due to screening and treatment disparities.) But everyone is at risk for this type of cancer, and the numbers are telling: Colorectal cancer remains the second leading cause of cancer-related deaths in the US. And it's not just older folks. There's been a distressing trend of colorectal cancer in a younger demographic—people under fifty. Which is why "forty-five is the new fifty" when it comes to screening now (if you have no family history; if you do, start at forty). People need to know: This is a cancer that is preventable through screening and easily treatable when detected early—up to 90 percent of patients diagnosed early are cured. But you need to participate in that screening and take advantage of the incredible technologies we have today to prevent this disease. Screening helps us do two things—it helps us detect and remove precancerous polyps before they turn into cancer, and it helps us find colon and rectal cancers at an early stage when they are still curable. Many other cancers are likewise very curable today, but only if you're on your game and getting screened routinely and on time.

Q. Are you a fan of at-home test kits like Cologuard?

A. Absolutely. I like to encourage people to do what's easy for them. Cologuard is just one of seven approved strategies to get screened for colorectal cancer. These strategies include stool-based and noninvasive tests that you can do at home like the fecal immunochemical test (FIT) and Cologuard, and more invasive procedures like colonoscopy. So there's no excuse; there's an option for everyone. If one of the at-home stool-based tests is what it takes to get you in the door for initial screening, do it. If it comes back positive, of course then you must go for the traditional colonoscopy as that is the only way we can say for certain that you do not have precancerous polyps or cancer. Talk to your doctor about the different options, discuss the pros and cons of them, and find what's best for you. Cancer screenings are critical to detect disease early. We like to say: The best test is the test that gets done!

Q. How are we going to close the gap between those who have access to high-quality healthcare and individuals from under-resourced settings?

A. I'm passionate about my work to address health disparities. Each person should have the opportunity to have the highest level of health, which begins with screening and prevention. But the reality is that many people live in a medical desert—over 84 million Americans live in places where there's a shortage of primary care professionals. It can be difficult to see a doctor even when you're insured. Such a reality is why I'm a coleader of Stand Up to Cancer's Colorectal Cancer Health Equity Dream Team. We are bringing screening tests to the medically underserved communities around the country. There's a lot of work to be done, and not just in my specialty but across all cancers. With better awareness, access, policies, and advocacy, we can build a healthier tomorrow.

A Call from Harvard

With our work in the Obama initiative, I was learning about all cancers. I was seeing the consistencies in the challenges and the opportunities. It was clear that our models in myeloma could benefit so many organizations and patients. And with Nicole in Uganda and David in college, there was time to grow a bit. In time, my work would transition, too.

In the fall of 2015, I received a call from the dean of Harvard Business School (HBS). They had been gifted a $20M grant to accelerate precision medicine by building collaborations and business models that could drive the field forward. I would now become a faculty co-chair of the Harvard Business School Kraft Precision Medicine Accelerator. This move, however, meant I needed someone new to come in and run the MMRF—someone eminently qualified, someone I really trusted, someone who knew the staff, the board, and the key donors. An individual who knew how to run a growing team and stay true to the mission of accelerating cures. I decided that someone should be Paul and the board agreed. And while I thought that decision made perfect sense at the time, several trusted advisors warned me of the difficulties of spouses working together. Paul understood how important this was to me. He agreed to take the job.

I was excited to collaborate closely with Paul after these years of working apart, but it did come with challenges. It's hard for founders to let go and we had two very different management styles. In hindsight, perhaps the decision was in the best interest of myeloma patients but not in our best interest personally.

Being officially invested with accelerating cures across cancers and all diseases at HBS, while still driving the same mission in myeloma with Paul, only fueled my relentless drive. Over the years, I was constantly on the road racing back and forth to Boston. On the ride up, I'd be focused on everything we were doing at Harvard—convening high-level meetings with the best-in-class leaders across the entire oncology ecosystem, addressing the need for new models and approaches. It blew me away how much we could get incredibly smart people to share ideas and shave time off efforts in precision medicine. Driving back home, I'd be thinking how to bring some of the innovative ideas like new venture approaches, exciting platform trials, or direct-to-patient efforts back to the MMRF. The work at HBS was new and exciting, and I was fearless in my efforts to now change the system for all cancer patients. But having two "part-time" jobs with a three-hour commute was tougher than I thought. And then the real crisis hit. Paul and I were traveling together when we started getting texts from both Nicole and David. Our schedule was full and we were focused on our last day of meetings.

"You guys better get on your flight back," read one text. "Everything is shutting down," read another.

Step 12

Protect Your Family

How Do I Prevent Disease from the Start?

If we didn't know before, the COVID crisis showed us all that prevention starts with you. The actions you take have a direct impact on your ability to stay healthy. For people who are immunocompromised, either from cancer, another health condition, or age, taking preventative actions become even more important. Even urgent.

Just as there's an urgency with illness, there's an urgency in prevention. Your journey—and hopefully this book—has shown you how diseases impact you and yours. You have witnessed the issues from a medical, emotional, and financial perspective. And you don't wish this to be repeated on those you love. The good news is modern medicine has a lot to offer beyond treatments, and the opportunities grow in number every day. Every year, we gain new knowledge about how nutrition and lifestyle habits can extend life and give you more time to enjoy healthy years. Every year, new technologies emerge that can detect disease earlier and better vaccinate against it.

But as they say, time is of the essence. Don't delay. Talk with those close to you, especially the next generation, your children. They may be years from any health challenges, but prevention always begins today. Now is the time to share the many ways we can protect ourselves from difficult diseases. Now is the time to establish healthy habits for ourselves and for those around us. After all, the best way to cure any disease is to not get it. The next best way is to find it as early as possible so it can be treated. In today's world of fast-moving science, the promise of new therapies and diagnostics is exploding. We saw it firsthand during the COVID crisis. And we need to keep learning from it.

Lessons from COVID

The phones at the MMRF rang nonstop once the pandemic was officially declared. Patients were calling both me personally and Paul at the foundation's helm. They had so many unanswered questions. And while Paul and I had agreed he would stay at the MMRF until we identified the next CEO (which we had), he felt responsible to get the team through this challenging time. He went to the office every morning at the same time he always did, met our CFO (the only other person coming in), refocused the team in a virtual world, made sure the systems would support everyone, and conducted weekly Zoom calls to stay in close touch. Together, we worked with our chief medical officer to answer the endless reasonable questions we were getting on an hourly basis.

Every patient was different, with vast and diverse needs:

"Should I go to the hospital for treatment?" (Only if you have to because you're more likely to be exposed outside of your home. See if your clinician can switch you to an oral drug for now.)

"What is happening with the clinical trial I am in? Should I stay in it?" (Yes, if they can find a way to mail you the drug or get it to you safely.)

"How should I stay in touch with my doctor?" (Ask for telemedicine and make sure it's covered.)

Then came the countless questions on the diagnostic testing:

"Do I want the antigen test, the antibody test? Where am I going to get it? How can I get it? When can I get it?"

And finally, "Which vaccine to get—Moderna? Pfizer? Astra Zen-eca?"

Nothing could be scarier than having a history of cancer or being an active cancer patient knowing there's a life-threatening microbe on the prowl, in this case a virus. Patients were rightfully terrified. The pandemic taught us important lessons about general preven-tion, such as the value in handwashing and mask-wearing, staying home when not feeling well, testing for the virus, and being mind-ful of the air quality and individuals in proximity. We all suddenly became much more attentive to people's health status, age, and vul-nerabilities. But for cancer patients, the bar to clear to protect our-selves and our families was much higher. Healthy people could avoid hospitals and doctor's appointments for a while, and they avoided cancer screenings, too. (In April 2020, screenings for breast, colon, prostate, and lung cancers were lower by 85 percent, 75 percent, 74 percent, and 56 percent, respectively*; this likely means more can-cer diagnoses for years to come.) Throughout the changing waves of the pandemic, cancer patients had to figure out how to manage risk. Some patients made difficult decisions about delaying certain treatments or putting off getting the COVID vaccine itself because of their cancer treatments. And being both high-risk for breast can-cer and potentially high-risk for COVID (as myeloma weakens your immune system), I had my own difficult decisions to make. I decided not to miss a screening, but I would take precautions.

Beyond thinking about my own screenings and health, Paul and I strived to make sure our family remained safe from the moment the pandemic was declared and the death rates started to climb. Like everyone else who could stay at home, isolation set in as we distanced ourselves from other family members, including my mom and Karen's

---

* See: Debra Patt, et al. "Impact of COVID-19 on Cancer Care: How the Pandemic Is Delaying Cancer Diagnosis and Treatment for American Seniors," *JCO Clinical Cancer Informatics* 4 (November 2020): 1059–1071.

family. Serenity came most when we were able to just get out and walk around our neighborhood. David and I started fostering dogs, which meant we were constantly taking them (and ourselves) out for much-needed walks. Bonnie, Bridget, Tiffany, and I became our own COVID pod, walking endlessly whenever and wherever we could.

But over time it became clear that this crisis was going to drag on until we got a vaccine.

As David expected, the hiatus that sports teams had to take meant his newly found job at NBC Sports was in jeopardy. Six months into the pandemic, the prediction became reality and he was out of work. In a smart move, David switched to online courses to stay busy and landed a job selling diagnostics. It turned out to be one of the best moves he ever made. Nicole had taken her incredible experience in Uganda and turned it into an application to Harvard Business School herself. She had extended her stay beyond the one year in maternal health and started her own nonprofit there called ACT (an acronym for Acrobatics Circus Troupe). The mission of the organization was to use performance art to support the children of Katwe, an under-resourced community in the capital city of Kampala. ACT continues today and became a critical resource for awareness and education during the pandemic. Now here she was as a second-year at HBS, sitting in her apartment doing classes online. Like every other student, she made the best of it.

When the vaccine became available, Paul and I ran to the pharmacy. It was an incredible, celebratory moment for us just to feel a bit of relief. As leaders at the MMRF, we felt equally responsible for the staff and the patients we served. And as more questions came in, we continually did the research to arrive at answers.

Dr. Ebright remained the person we trusted in terms of what tests to do and what vaccines to take. She was always available on telemedicine when we were dealing with potential infections, a scary situation given my history. And while we were all being told to stay out of the hospitals, she was the one person reminding us not to miss any critical screenings. By now, she knew Nicole, David, and me very well. She had worked with me to make sure Nicole and David received the right vaccines for their age, including the one for HPV. And she pushed me on the shingles vaccine. My visits with Dr. Ebright also reminded me not to miss my screenings with Dr. Port, even as COVID was surging again with a new omicron mutation that seemed to defy the vaccine.

It was a little more than a week before Christmas in 2021, full COVID protocols in force, when I went in for my annual MRI and Dr. Port first detected the earliest sign of breast cancer. "We saw something. . . . A spot . . . Could be nothing. . . . Let's not take any chances. . . . We should go in and check it out. . . ."

I didn't panic. I was a good patient at this point and knew the routine. My situation called for annual MRIs so the doctor could see the tissue better. Benign spots often showed up. The previous year she'd performed a needle biopsy on a questionable spot that turned out to be nothing to worry about.

"We found something right at the same spot as before, and it looks bigger," she said. "I'd say there's a ten, maybe twenty percent chance it's cancer."

I let her go on about next steps. She wanted to take a closer look with a surgical biopsy because it was too hard to maneuver needle biopsies on my flat chest. "I don't trust needle biopsies on you anymore," she said. "And I need you to hang around for some more imaging today so we get a new baseline on you."

I agreed to the imaging and we began the process of scheduling, planning, and filling out forms for the surgery in January. I'd been through this possibility before and had learned not to sound any foreboding bells while I didn't know anything for sure. It was normal for me to compartmentalize by now, especially over the holidays, and wait until I could undergo more tests. Part of me had known this was coming. It was why I was doing the screenings. As I had learned, the best way to prevent cancer is to understand your risk and find it early, when it can be cured.

Make Prevention Primary

Overnight, COVID made the entire country aware of prevention. Nicole and David were petrified of getting me, Paul, Karen, or my mom sick. Yet we still wanted to see each other. I was blown away by their mask compliance and tenacious testing. If there was the slightest risk they'd been in contact with someone, they stayed in their apartments.

When any of us did feel sick, we relied on Dr. Ebright and the world of telemedicine. Folding Nicole and David into her practice was one of the best moves I'd made. We waited way too long to move them from the pediatrician to an internist who would focus on their adult needs. It honestly took my seeing David sitting in the waiting room at nearly six feet tall with five-year-olds before I caught on.

Both Nicole and David are hugely aware of our lousy genes. All it took was one ancestry project they did in high school to see how many of their grandparents had passed away from cancer. They waste no time doing research when a symptom emerges. I don't blame them. But even more importantly, as they get older, they have a clinician who is highly aware of their risks and keeps them on their game. Dr. Ebright knows our entire family history. She knows how to advise them moving forward. She keeps copious records for them in case they move and need to switch their care. Most importantly, she stays on top of the new methods of diagnostic testing.

Over time, and likely in Nicole's and David's early lifetimes, we will begin to see diagnostic testing in cancer that looks nothing like today's. Companies are already emerging that can pick up potential cancer DNA through a simple blood test. And as these tests get refined with fewer false positives, it will be important that they are accessible and covered by insurance. This technology is something the next generation must be aware of and pursue.

The best way not to get cancer is to prevent it. The best way to protect your family is to share your medical history and let them know their risk. It will allow them to work with their primary care doctor to focus on good habits and prevention.

STEP 12: PROTECT YOUR FAMILY

WTDs

Find a Good Primary Care Doctor
X Know the types of primary care doctors
X Know how to choose them
X Know the vaccines they can provide

Stay on Top of the Latest Preventive Science
X Multicancer early-detection tests (MCEDs)
X Genetic testing

Model Good Health Habits
X Don't use tobacco
X Protect yourself from the sun
X Maintain a healthy body weight and be physically active
X Eat a healthy diet
X Minimize alcohol intake
X Practice good sleep hygiene and mindfulness

WTD 1: Find a Good Primary Care Doctor

According to the American Association of Family Practice Physicians (AAFP), "a primary care physician is a specialist in family medicine, general internal medicine, or general pediatrics who provides definitive care to the undifferentiated patient at the first point of contact, and takes continuing responsibility for providing the patient's comprehensive care." Bottom line is, PCPs not only help you in acute situations where you feel sick, they're your partner in preventing you from getting sick in the first place.

✓ *Know the types of primary care doctors*

There is more than one kind of primary care doctor. It's important to understand the right one for you.

→ **Internal medicine doctors**: These doctors only care for adults. They are called internists and are trained to treat both simple and complex conditions. They are able to follow the patient from early adulthood through old age. Internal medicine doctors may also be trained in a subspecialty like gastroenterology, rheumatology, or cardiology.

→ **Family medicine doctors**: These doctors care for your entire family. They often understand your family history and, if treating your entire family, can provide helpful, personalized care. They are trained to work with all ages and understand a broad range of diseases.

→ **General practitioners**: These doctors treat adults, adolescents, and children. General practice doctors may choose to practice family medicine, but family medicine is an actual specialty.

✓ *Know how to choose them*

Choosing your primary care doctor can be one of the most important healthcare decisions you'll ever make. The decision is personal, but there are a number of considerations:

→ **Make sure they are in-network**: It's best to ask your insurance company, Medicare, or Medicaid for names that are in network. Again, you don't want to pay out-of-pocket expenses for someone you will see on a regular basis.

→ **Ask for referrals**: It's always good to ask your other doctors for a recommendation. They often work together in a hospital system and hear the good and bad of their colleagues. Your friends can provide input as well.

→ **Go visit the office**: As we discussed in previous chapters, just make sure you feel comfortable in the setting. Was it easy to schedule the appointment? Is the receptionist helpful? The nursing staff? How long did you wait? Were all your questions answered and the answers easy to understand?

✓ *Know the vaccines they can provide*

Vaccines are one of the most powerful tools we have to prevent disease. Work with your PCP to discuss every vaccine and preventive measure for every stage of your and your family's life. If you have concerns or questions, you should discuss them openly with your doctor.

WTD 2: Stay on Top of the Latest Preventive Science

The science of preventive medicine is advancing at incredible rates. Stay up to date with your vaccines and screenings and ask your primary care doctor about every new vaccine and diagnostic test you come across. Here are some of the new preventive tools that are on the horizon and worth keeping an eye on.

✓ *Multicancer early-detection tests (MCEDs)*

According to the American Cancer Society, MCEDs might be useful in preventing cancer deaths. While we communicated proven screening tests in Step 11, 70 percent of all cancer deaths come from cancers for which there is no proven screening. As of today, there are a number of MCEDs, but they are not yet approved by the FDA. Instead, they fall under the category of CLIA (Clinical Laboratory Improvement Act) regulations, meaning your doctor can order them on your behalf. If you ask your doctor about an MCED, be sure to confirm the cost and coverage. MCEDs will likely be used in higher-risk people and supplement the screenings noted earlier.

✓ *Genetic testing*

There is extensive work being done today to identify new genetic biomarkers for a range of diseases. Today, companies like 23andMe offer direct-to-consumer genetic testing where you can send in a saliva sample and find out whether you have a genetic predisposition for ten different diseases, including the BRCA gene for breast cancer. The number of diseases will only grow in time as genetic biomarker research advances. If you believe like I do that information is power, you can use services like this to learn about your risks and take steps to reduce them such as increased screening or other interventions. Whole genome sequencing, which provides a much more detailed record of your DNA, will become increasingly available and economical in the future. According to Eric Lefkofsky, founder of one of the companies that provides genomic sequencing (Tempus), "In the future, whole genome sequencing will happen when you're born and you can be followed throughout your life."

WTD 3: Model Good Health Habits

This seems obvious, I know, but modeling healthy habits should be your first defense in preventing disease. In my life, I prioritize exercise, sleep, eating healthily, and maintaining relationships. According to the National Institutes of Health, "Seven out of ten deaths in the United

States are the result of chronic diseases, which for many people can be prevented by eating well, staying physically active, avoiding tobacco use and excessive drinking, and getting regular health screenings." The same applies to cancer. The Mayo Clinic website provides a number of tips to reduce the risk of cancer:

✓ **Don't use tobacco**
It's important to stay away from both smoking and chewing tobacco. Smoking, or being near secondhand smoke, has been associated with cancer of the lung, mouth, throat, voice box, pancreas, bladder, cervix, and kidney.

✓ **Protect yourself from the sun**
The Mayo site reminds us that skin cancer is one of the most preventable cancers out there. Use sunscreen, stay out of the sun (especially at midday), and don't use a tanning bed.

✓ **Maintain a healthy body weight and be physically active**
Being at a healthy weight for your body type may lower the risk of breast, prostate, lung, colon, and kidney cancer. The Mayo site recommends thirty minutes of physical activity per day.

✓ **Eat a healthy diet**
No surprises here. The site recommends eating plenty of fruits and vegetables and other foods from plant sources like whole grains and beans. Stay away from processed sugars and processed meats. The Mediterranean diet, focused on olive oil, plant-based foods, and fish, is recommended.

✓ **Minimize alcohol intake**
Alcohol is increasingly shown to be a big risk factor for cancer. If you consume alcohol, practice moderation.

✓ *Practice good sleep hygiene and mindfulness*

I've already spoken about the role of good sleep hygiene and meditation in treating cancer. But good sleep and mindfulness can also play a role in overall health and wellbeing. Good sleep is important for maintaining a robust immune system, reducing stress, and promoting overall wellness, while poor sleep has been linked to increased inflammation, hormonal imbalance, and weight gain, all risk factors for various types of cancer. Mindfulness practices such as meditation can also help reduce stress, improve sleep, and potentially increase immune function.

IN CONVERSATION WITH MARK MCCLELLAN

former commissioner of the U.S. Food and Drug Administration and former administrator of the Centers for Medicare and Medicaid Services

Mark McClellan, MD, PhD, is not only a physician but also an economist who has addressed a wide range of health strategies and reforms in his role as director of Duke University's Margolis Center for Health Policy. He was pivotal in the US response to COVID, pushing for early tracking, testing, then prevention through vaccines to contain and combat the pandemic. His contributions ultimately helped our country reopen safely. I was curious to get his input on the parallels he's made between his experience handling the crisis of the pandemic and the cancer world.

Q. What prevention lessons from the COVID pandemic apply to oncology today?
A. First, during the early phase of the pandemic, we had to learn who was at most risk for serious illness and death: the elderly and people with underlying conditions. These are the same vulnerable populations for cancer because age is the biggest risk factor

for the disease, and older people are more likely to live with concomitant illness, too. Once you know where you stand on the spectrum of risk for a disease, you can then take precautionary steps to reduce your vulnerability. Secondly, the COVID crisis also taught us the importance of high-quality, reliable diagnostic testing that's easily accessible and covered (free). Same goes for cancer—you want to spot the problem as soon as possible when it's more treatable and less costly to overcome. And thirdly, the pandemic showed the power of prevention and practicing good hygiene—from washing hands often to getting good sleep. Similarly, the best way to manage cancer is to avoid developing it to begin with by practicing those anticancer habits.

Q. What's your best piece of advice for people who want to protect themselves from serious illness?
A.   Have a good primary care physician (PCP) that you like and who will be your partner and ally in all things healthcare related. This means having a trustworthy PCP who teaches health-promoting lifestyle habits—the importance of diet, exercise, and life-saving vaccines—and who stays updated with the latest technologies in prevention, including screenings and diagnostics. Your PCP is your ultimate guardrail against disease. The goal is to maintain optimal health to tip the scales in your favor when you get sick.

Q. How can we do better on the policy side?
A.   Policy reforms can address three critical needs in the delivery and economics of care: improving health equity to help more people gain affordable access; expanding coverage to lower overall costs to patients; and promoting better outcomes through a greater focus on prevention. Unfortunately, many Americans are unable to access the full spectrum of preventive strategies available today. This is precisely why we need leadership in the policy realm to address these delivery and economic challenges and

improve healthcare for everyone. You may not be in a position to reform policy directly, but you can have an impact through your voting practices and writing letters to your local members of Congress. No one should have to choose between what they need to stay healthy and what they can afford—from cutting-edge screening and diagnostic testing to treatment and beyond. This access is especially critical in the cancer world where you're up against time with a serious diagnosis, and the financial burden can be large.

❋

Another Christmas, Another January, Another Diagnosis

We celebrated Christmas Eve and Christmas Day as we always did— with my mom and the Andrewses. Despite the ongoing pandemic and huge rise in cases due to omicron, my family took the necessary precautions and checked all the traditional holiday boxes, including tolerating my awful cooking on Christmas Eve and playing the Fishbowl game that combines charades, Password, and Taboo. For us, with twentysomethings in the house, most answers were inappropriate but garnered lots of laughs. On Christmas morning, we woke up, Paul lit the fire, and we opened presents and made our usual breakfast. On the way to Karen's house, we stopped as always at Paul's parents' cemetery, knowing how much he still missed them. My mom was staying with us again and we were grateful for the time. She was over ninety years old now and every holiday with her held special meaning. Even though it was getting harder for her to get around and she'd had a stroke, she remained staunchly determined. And she never let me forget her final wishes. While Karen would be her executor, I had been her medical proxy. We'd taken hours to make sure I knew what she wanted when her final days came. Most importantly, her wish to die at home.

In January, Paul and I took our COVID tests and headed to Mt. Sinai for the surgical biopsy. When we went back for the biopsy's results, I had to go in alone due to the strict COVID restrictions. The
clinic was busy. Dr. Port rushed into the exam room, sat down with a
stack of papers—clearly my results—and got right to the point.

"The surgery looks great and the biopsy scar is healing perfectly.
But we have the pathology back on the tissue and you have a very
early form of breast cancer called DCIS."

My mind started to reel. Ductal carcinoma in situ (DCIS), I'd later
come to learn, refers to there being abnormal cells inside a milk duct
in my breast that have not spread to other tissues. DCIS is considered
the earliest form of breast cancer—stage zero. Still, it's cancer.

She continued in rapid-fire doctor speak, using terminology that
was everyday lingo in her domain. She quickly noted the cancer's
type, location, and margins.

"It's low grade and ER-positive—all good factors. It does mean
that moving forward, monitoring you, we need to look at every MRI
with a very close eye. With your history, it's likely we will continue
seeing things and will need to continue doing surgical biopsies. It
will be more visits, of course. There's no way around that. So, let's go
through all this again . . ."

I was a high-risk patient due to the radiation I'd undergone with
my myeloma. The words "DCIS" and "ER-positive" were somewhat
familiar thanks to my sister's journey. I could barely catch my breath
before she dived into options to consider for next steps.

"At a minimum, you will be on active surveillance using MRIs and
surgical biopsies," Port said, "but we do have to treat this. Let's go
through the options." Right off the bat, she said: "Mastectomy." (The
look on my face must have read *horror*.) "Lumpectomy with or without radiation or chemotherapy," she went on, adding that there were
additional tests they could do to see what was best. And then drug
regimens using anastrozole or tamoxifen—a world I also recognized
immediately.

"*That one* has done a number on my sister," I quickly interjected. Karen had chosen the drug route for her breast cancer, and it had not been an easy road. Port pointed out that my sister's diagnosis was different. DCIS was not Stage III breast cancer. While I could learn from Karen's case, it was not the same as mine.

Then came the list.

"See the medical oncologist," she said, reminding me that she's the *surgical* oncologist with her own bias. "See the radiation folks . . . even talk with other surgical oncologists. And, of course, talk to your sister. Take your time. You have time. Let's do what's right for you. I am here for you. You can call me anytime. I am going to do another MRI in three months and see you then at a minimum."

Port handed me a piece of paper with the names of the other doctors to consult. Swirling always at the back of my mind was the thought that I *don't have time for this*. I can't put my family through more cancer again. I could see the calendar filling with appointments, days off work, mileage, support. It was all too much. *WTF?* reverberated in my head yet again as I remembered the beat-up calendar from so many years ago, and the many appointments that filled it.

Clearly, I had some homework to do, and it was up to me to get the best information. I left in a daze as I checked out, exited the building, and found Paul parked illegally out front waiting for me.

"How'd it go?" he asked as soon as I slid into the car.

"I have breast cancer but it's early," I said. He looked shocked, barely able to process the news, and I told him again.

"I just didn't see this coming," Paul said.

Once we were on our way, I explained to him that I had options. But we both went a bit quiet. As I carefully punched "DCIS" into my phone in search of some online resources, a text from Nicole came in promptly: "How was it? What did they say?" I called her right back.

"It's going to be fine, Nicole. I do have breast cancer but it is *so* early. I honestly feel a bit fortunate, like perhaps I dodged a bullet here. Do you understand what I'm saying?"

"Are you sure you're telling me everything?" Nicole probed.

"I will let you read the reports, no problem," I said. Now she was old enough and I knew she just might take me up on that.

"I love you."

"Love you, too. I'll call David," I said, knowing she'd text him immediately upon hanging up. David's response was quintessential:

"You've got this, Mom." I would later learn that this diagnosis, now that he was an adult, was tougher on him. But in the weeks and months to come, he and his sweet girlfriend, Abby, would help get me through the surgeries and infections.

Days later, I knew it was time to tell my mom. I couldn't do it over the phone, so I drove to her farmhouse four hours away and we went to lunch. Her response was typical "Grammy." "Everyone gets breast cancer. You know how to do this. You'll get through it just fine," she said.

In her mind, she had watched me move through multiple myeloma, a blood cancer, for decades. And while she would never say she was proud of my work, as a former nurse, she knew the impact of my long days, constant travel, and pharma meetings. She had attended every major fundraising event, listening to each emotional speech I took weeks to craft in an effort to raise desperately needed funds. She knew how formidable I'd been to find new life-saving drugs that would help me and others. She, too, had seen my caregiving skills as a melanoma patient herself. It was my job to balance more treatments and surgeries with her quality of life. It was my job to find homecare so she could live in the house she loved. Even now, looking across the table at lunch while she ate her French fries (which she had ordered so I could take them off her plate), her face was again laced with stitches from more cancer surgeries. Her eye still drooped just a bit from the surgery she'd endured without a single complaint years before.

This was my mother—a woman hell-bent on not worrying her family. She wore her battle scars proudly. The situation was practically comical. I appreciated her levity but also knew that despite my not-so-serious breast cancer, I needed to make decisions. I needed to make contact with a host of people to personalize my own treatment going forward. I was calm and cool, but I wouldn't say I was collected yet.

I had done my research. I knew everything about DCIS. I had spoken with leaders in the field. The answers were not consistent, but they never are. I listened closely to those who had known me through myeloma. I listened closely to my primary care doctor. But it was the one statement I heard from the head of a breast cancer center that resonated most: "Kathy, you gave up your entire life, *decades* of your life, finding a cure for myeloma. In one surgical procedure, albeit a tough one, you can be cured. Why would you not do that now?" My decision was made.

My breast cancer was the chance to put everything I learned to the test. The twelve hard-learned steps that cured my myeloma emboldened me. And those steps would prove to work the second time around:

1. **Understand the Diagnosis:** I did the research, asked the right questions, and googled wisely.
2. **Meet the Specialists:** I met the doctors to fully understand my diagnosis and options.
3. **Rethink What Matters:** I went through my own reset: established my personal goals to inform my treatment decisions (opting to treat aggressively to be done with treatment and off the roller coaster as soon as possible).
4. **Make Your Action Plan:** I devised a plan (and adapted when things didn't go accordingly).
5. **Get the Right Team:** I curated the right medical team and kept them all informed.
6. **Get the Right Tests:** I got the critical tests to inform my treatment choices.

7. ***Get the Right Treatments:*** I made the treatment decision that was right for me.
8. ***Know the Right Trial:*** I didn't need a trial, but I used everything at my disposal (research, coordinating medical teams) to navigate the post-surgery complications.
9. ***Reset (Again):*** I underwent another personal reset having gotten through my cancer (more on this in a moment).
10. ***Recognize Your Caregivers:*** I leaned on my personal support team every step of the way, communicating clearly with them to get what I needed, and making sure they knew how much I appreciated their help.
11. ***Never Miss a Screening:*** I found the cancer early when it was curable by knowing my risk and undergoing the proper screenings.
12. ***Protect Your Family:*** I continue to focus on prevention and talking to my children.

The twelve steps worked . . . as best as any playbook can. But I was reminded in the process how humbling cancer can be. It's a formidable foe and even when you have the background to do it all right, you can still screw it up. It was hard to integrate the care between Dana-Farber for my myeloma and Mt. Sinai for my breast cancer. There were times in the ERs when I was too sick to talk and wished I'd had everything written out in one place. And managing coverage was a nightmare. I actually ended up paying a significant amount out of pocket because I missed that step on the paperwork in the surgeon's office.

But what I've learned along the way, what finally hit me in the face in real-life wake-up-call Technicolor was this: How you save your life from cancer isn't enough. You have to think about how you live your life, as well. The people who know me are likely surprised how this playbook asks you to keep sitting down and evaluating your life during your cancer journey. They will tell you, that's not Kathy. She's direct, brutally direct, and fast. Check that box, do it now, don't wait for tomorrow. They would be right: I was fearless. But as I learned writing this book, being fearless comes with a cost. That's what I want to share with you now, so you can learn from my mistakes. Here goes.

PART 4

The Final Reset

EPILOGUE

My Final Reset

When I started writing this book, I thought it would be the last chapter in my cancer story. I had been fighting cancer for twenty-five years, first taking on a broken medical system to save my own life, then working to change that system to save countless others. There was no second cancer diagnosis in my life, no new pathogen to battle. It was time for me to step back, time to retreat from the front lines and reflect on everything I had learned along the way so I could share it with you.

My process of self-reflection, what turned out to be a soul-searching examination of my life, began with my journals. I pulled the twenty-five books off the shelf and stacked them on my desk; twenty-five journals for twenty-five years I wasn't expected to live. Each one a different size, a different color—forest green, royal purple, bubblegum pink—reflecting Nicole's or David's favorite color of that year. Each one having sat unopened since the day it was completed, a window into fears long since erased, hidden truths waiting to be exhumed. The unopened pile spoke volumes about my life, fiercely driving forward, never stopping to revisit the past. It was time for the excavation to begin.

I took the first journal off the top of the pile and stared at the orange sunflower on the cover. Is that why I bought it? Sunflowers are symbols for happiness and resilience, known for their tall, strong stems and ability to thrive in difficult conditions, flowers always turning to face the sun. Was I thinking that at the time? I saw myself back in that Borders bookstore and relived my worst fear, that I wouldn't live to see Nicole go to kindergarten.

I opened the front cover of the journal and read the inscription: *To Paul and Nicole, who make life worth living. . . .*

I then turned the blank page and these were the words that popped out at me: *multiple myeloma—big words for a little girl but they mean Mommy has a disease that she must fight. . . .*

Page two, I was already moving from fatal to fearless. What helped me overcome my fear? What made me fight like hell? The answer was Nicole and Paul, and just a couple journals later, Nicole's brother, David.

Journal by journal I relived my last twenty-five years. Being fearless didn't end with my remission. I would go on to raise half a billion dollars for research at the MMRF and triple life expectancy for people with myeloma. I would take every call from every patient and doctor for decades—at any hour of the day, including weekends. I would give my life to the cause, believing I got up every day doing what others could only dream of doing. Curing cancer—how could you have a nobler cause? More purpose? And we were doing it surprisingly well. So well, in fact, that we were the model for every other cancer and disease institute. I had started the journey with good intentions, the best, and felt an incredible accountability to the broader cancer community. But as was painfully self-evident in reading my journals, without boundaries, being fearless came with a cost.

My transplant during Karen's divorce. Paul selling his company so we could move to Connecticut, then stepping in at the MMRF so I could move on to bigger battles. Constant testing and treatments when David and Nicole needed me most. Had I paid enough attention to the people who really mattered, the very people who gave me the will to survive in the first place?

Keep our family safe and happy. Those were the words of my primary want, the words I wrote down in that very first journal. I should have plastered that want everywhere and across every page on every journal thereafter. Now, twenty-five years later, sitting down to write this book, I took out a blank sheet of paper. What do I want now?

That was when I was diagnosed with breast cancer.

My decision would be preordained when I closed my last journal. My fears this time wouldn't be about the cancer—I had caught it plenty early. My fears would be about what the cancer would do to Nicole and to David, and to Paul and Karen. How could I make it easier this time? Less burdensome on everyone? I went back to see Dr. Port very confident in my decision. Double mastectomy would be the fastest and most direct path to a cure. She warned me it was a tough surgery and to brace for the pain and discomfort, as well as potential complications. I told her I was ready; I was doing it for the ability to get off the ride and finally, in my sixties, begin believing that cancer was not going to continue dominating my life or the lives of my family. No more treatments after this. No more testing. Perhaps just some real normalcy. She explained that there was no bad decision here. There was only the right decision for me. And it was mine to make.

Cancer Is Humbling

Dr. Port gave me the name of the best plastic surgeon she knew. The two of them would pass the baton in the operating room as she removed all the breast tissue and he prepared me for reconstruction. As I began to get ready for the surgery and organize my schedule, I called my friend Tiffany. Coincidentally, she had been through this exact process with the exact same doctors. When she had been diagnosed with breast cancer two years earlier, she'd come to me for recommendations on doctors and I had recommended Dr. Port. Her experience had gone well and she was happy to share every detail. Over coffee (and a few beers, too), Tiffany walked me through the toughest part— the surgery itself. Her advice was invaluable as was her friendship.

My breast cancer journey started with a delay and a detour. I should have known I was going to be in trouble right then. Paul was ready to drive me to the hospital for the much-awaited surgery. Nicole and David were both home to help take care of me. They'd called in their favors at work to make sure they were available. My friends were on call for whatever was needed. Karen would be up to visit as soon as I got home. It was "go time" and my team was ready. And then the morning of surgery, Dr. Port called to cancel. Despite feeling fine, my pre-op COVID test had come back positive. Now I was delayed by weeks because the surgical suite was still catching up from the COVID pandemic. There was no space to fit me in.

Finally, we "re-did" it all, the paperwork, the tests, the team adjusting their work schedules and calls. Paul drove me to the hospital and waited for Dr. Port to call and let him know that everything had gone well. He stayed with me there off and on for days until it was time for me to come home. He helped me with the drains, the bandages, the meds. Nicole would help me bathe and watch countless, mindless episodes of *Love Island*. David and Abby cooked the most amazing meals and walked the dogs. We were okay.

Until it was time to take the bandages off. I had noticed some pink sneaking through the bottom of the bandages of the left breast. The plastic surgeon kept a very calm poker face, but it was clear I had an infection. The skin had not closed properly. As a perfectionist, he was calm but not pleased. I was back to another delay. Nothing could happen except to hope that the skin would heal and antibiotics would take away the infection. We spent weeks in this space—no movement forward. Delay, delay. Keep driving to New York. And back. In rush-hour traffic.

Then the call came from our sweet mother's caregiver. "Your mom fell. I think she had another stroke. She just left her farmhouse in an ambulance." With my bandages still on, I packed all my antibiotics and creams and raced to the hospital trying desperately to beat the traffic, with the Waze app throwing off over four hours of driving time. At first, we thought this was another mini-stroke and our miracle mom would do a few weeks in PT/OT and be right back at it. But one mini-stroke became another and the blood in her brain was seeping. In a matter of hours, she started to lose the ability to move her limbs, then her hands, and then her speech. On the way, I called Karen, who had gotten there in record time. Together we knew: Get her home. I kept hearing our mother's voice: "Please, Kathy, you have one job, please don't let me die in a hospital."

Yet here I was, trying to beat a system that wasn't allowing me to get her home quickly. I did not know the world of palliative or hospice care. I was racing to find the right team to sign off. We all knew she was dying, but there were protocols: tubes to be moved, medications to administer, hospice packs, and hospital beds to be delivered.

I called Paul and the kids to tell them to drive as fast as possible to say goodbye. It was torture. This was the only grandparent Nicole and David had ever known. We were relieved when the ambulance delivered her to the farmhouse she loved almost as much as she loved the beach. But for all our brushes with death, and my years of working with myeloma patients, Karen and I had never actually watched anyone die. We contacted our brothers, our mom's friends, and urged them to come and say goodbye. While she couldn't speak, she could hear everyone.

But days turned into weeks, and our mom continued to struggle. She had mouth sores, the start of bed sores, and her organs were failing ever so slowly; it was so hard to get her comfortable. When hospice came in once each morning to help with the sheets and bathing, we tried to learn every detail. The hardest part of it all was being the keeper of the drugs. I would look at Karen each time I tried to up the morphine but then feel badly knowing hospice was coming in to measure it. I didn't want her to suffer but I didn't want to go too far. But the labored breathing, the anxiety, the waiting, all of it was unbearable. I kept apologizing to Mom while Karen would tell her funny stories and play hymns that they both liked.

It was Mother's Day when we woke up, still in disbelief that she had made it through another night. She always hated Mother's Day, saying motherhood itself was the greatest gift, no need for cards or flowers. We prayed all day at her bedside. We hugged her, told her for the hundredth time how much we loved her. We fell asleep at eleven that night, and by one a.m. she was gone. We have no idea if she died on Mother's Day or the next day.

We called hospice and they came to us in the darkness of the night. The nurse pronounced our mom dead and then asked us to bathe her. It was one of the hardest yet beautiful things we've ever done. She then said it was time to place her in her favorite comfy outfit to go to the funeral home. At five a.m. the funeral home arrived and did all they could to protect us from watching our incredible mom be wheeled out in a black leather bag on a gurney. Nobody really prepares you for this. And everyone dies differently. Karen and I took solace knowing we did our best and we did it together.

We spent the rest of the morning with our mom's caregiver and best friend, revisiting every story. Karen started on the obituary while I began framing the eulogy. We had so many details to cover, from the program to the headstone to the death certificates. We drove back to Connecticut in our separate cars, but I kept her license plate in front of me the entire way. I couldn't leave her. We had just been through so much together, things we thought nobody could ever understand.

Our mom's funeral was exactly what she would have wanted. It was in her tiny Presbyterian church with a minister who adored her. At ninety-two, she only had so many surviving friends, but she would have been pleased by the turnout. Paul, ever the master speechwriter, had helped me with the eulogy. JJ, David, and Tyler served as her pallbearers and Nicole and Katy were the greeters. It poured when we headed to the gravesite, but she was finally with Dad, happy and at rest. The reception was filled with laughter, cocktails, and friendship. I will remain so grateful for every friend who drove the four hours there, to the middle of nowhere. It was a poignant reminder of what's really important in life.

When we'd finally made it home, I looked in the mirror. I was emotionally and physically drained. And yes, still infected. Breast cancer was going to be a very long haul. We went back to the surgeon, who decided it was time to close the small problematic wound in his office. As Paul and I left that day, the doctor's voice was clear: "If you get a temperature over 101, here is my cell phone. Call me immediately." He watched while I put his name and number in my contacts. Little did I know how much I'd use that number.

Just days later, the Thursday leading up to Memorial Day weekend (six months since Dr. Port had first raised the possibility of a diagnosis), I finished a call and let Nicole know I wasn't feeling well, that I was taking a nap. She told me to take my phone with me and text her if I felt worse. Thirty minutes later, I texted her and she came running in. Quickly shoving the thermometer in my mouth, we called the doctor's office. They explained the surgeon was in the OR but they wanted to get a picture to him ASAP. As had been the case all along with this infection, I'd been sending daily photos of the left breast his way. With my fever now over 102 and a very pink photo in hand, they said drive to Mt. Sinai now. Nicole called Paul but he didn't pick up. I was hedging, just too sick to face the ninety minutes into the city on a holiday. She brought David in for reinforcement as they warmed the car up and got me going. Paul did make it, racing me to the hospital as quickly as possible and sitting with me in the ER. You never want to enter a teaching hospital over a holiday weekend.

I don't remember the ride and I barely remember the ER. I do remember testing positive for COVID again. I recall the ER staff and surgical residents debating how much of my fever, chills, and uncontrollable shaking were COVID versus something starting to look like sepsis. I was reminded of the days of transplant lying on the frozen sheets hoping to die. It was all topped off with my response to the vancomycin being pumped into me too quickly—a phenomenon known as Red Man's reaction. I honestly couldn't breathe. I had never experienced it before. Paul was screaming for help at this point. I don't know what I would have done if he had not been by my side. A huge ER on a holiday weekend is not the place to be alone.

As my surgeon arrived and studied all the labs, it was clear he needed to go in and remove the infected expander. The surgery took place at midnight. The surgeon urged Paul to go home because he would not be able to see me. I got to my room at four a.m. and stayed for four days on IV antibiotics. The peak of the roller coaster, the one I'd never wanted to be on. I was miserable, thinking I'd ruined yet another holiday weekend. While continued infections like this are rare, the new expander didn't take, and the scarring on my left breast remained pink. Every day I sent a photo to the surgeon. Every day he said "sit tight." Weeks passed.

Trying desperately to keep some normalcy, and knowing we had plans for July Fourth weekend with our family and friends, we kept it on the schedule. Tiffany and Bridget both came to help as their kids would be staying with us. David and Nicole warned their friends in advance that I wouldn't be myself (and not to hug me). My time was spent trying to look normal and happy while I went back up to my room to take my temperature, take naps, and send photos to the surgeon. The scars were a constant reminder of what I was still putting my family through. Another holiday ruined. On the final day, the surgeon asked Paul and me to drive back in so he could see me in person. He decided to do another surgery, take the expander out, and have me sit and do nothing for at least three months with no clear plan in sight.

The knot in my stomach was just like the cancer knot. How was I going to go back to my family, my friends, and ask for MORE help? More TIME. As I sat with my journals, the truth hit me hard: In healing my cancer, in working to heal everyone else's cancer, I was hurting the people I love the most. I was expecting too much. And now there was no light at the end of the tunnel.

Fatal to Fearless

One Saturday morning when I was at my lowest, the doorbell rang. There was Bonnie with a big cup of Starbucks coffee. She hugged me, knowing my radio silence signaled that something was truly bothering me. We sat on the stoop for over an hour talking. She knew my faults better than anyone and was not afraid to call me out on them—how even my closest friends had to schedule appointments through my assistant, how I was always on the phone even when we were together, how the great cancer-curing mission of Kathy Giusti always took priority. She also knew that people could change and shared her own personal struggle that led her to seek help and make shifts in her own life. I had known the story at the 20,000-foot level but this was different. I had incredible respect for all the hard work she did to get back on track. Bonnie became my new North Star. She had been beside me every step of the way, and would now stay beside me, encouraging me, coaching me, keeping me focused on the endgame of getting my priorities straight. Even in my sixties, it was not too late to change. Thank you, Bonnie.

I started thinking more deeply about the cost of cancer on loved ones and how I could repair what was broken. I read endless pieces on relationships and interpersonal communication. I walked our foster-fail dog Lola every morning listening to podcasts on the same. Who knew all this stuff was out there? Not me, apparently. For all the times I'd sat down and googled medical information, immersing myself into learning about the body and how it functions, I'd never once thought to learn about this touchy-feely stuff. I was astonished that I found it fascinating. I was a curious student and immersed myself in it, taking quizzes, workshops, doing one-hour sessions, you name it.

I was never a writer. I began writing that very first day of my puzzling myeloma diagnosis out of deep necessity. I didn't know another way to tell Nicole and Paul how much I loved them, a way to share the memories of our brief future together. A journal would be something they could read, and along with the endless photos and videos Paul took, a way to catch glimpses of a fun sunny day, a contagious laugh, a hug so tight you could barely breathe. In those early days, I was facing my mortality directly. The statistics were indisputable. Multiple myeloma was a death sentence with no funding and no drugs in the pipeline. It wasn't *if* I would die, it was *when*. And from what I could tell, it was three years.

We can all ask ourselves what we would do if we were told we were going to die, but it's impossible to answer until you experience it firsthand. The twenty-five journals stacked on my bookshelf were intended to be a gift for my family, but I lived, and they became an extraordinary gift to me, and hopefully, to you. The experience of referring to them in writing this book, reading back every single handwritten word and between every line, gave me the most beautiful, joyful, loving, embarrassing, shameful, guilt-ridden memories and insights you can imagine. Twenty-five years' worth. I got to revisit my life through those journals and rethink how I wanted to live now; it was equal parts awesome and heartbreaking, inspirational and instructive. Yes, it was all right in front of me. What I did right, what I did wrong, and what I didn't do at all.

Three years to live is an interesting time frame. It's just enough time to get a few things done but not enough time to see them through. I became determined to get shit done as fast and as perfectly as I could. Being fearless took over and allowed me to accomplish the unthinkable. When one thing worked, I found and chased the next. Now, there was more to do with the same twenty-four hours in a day and the total 26,280 hours I had left. Move, just move, keep moving.

Fearlessness saved my life. It taught me to be intensely curious and rapidly immerse myself in new knowledge. Yes, I knew the healthcare system from my work in the pharmaceutical industry. But my window seat as a patient gave me a whole new perspective of how screwed up it really was and still is. In record time, I learned every nook and cranny of the system. I noted every flaw and built a work-around. In days, I knew more about my disease than some of the doctors I was seeing. In weeks, I had built the best medical team I could find. In months, I started the MMRF with Karen's legal skills and Paul's donation. The first grants we funded immediately brought new scientists to the field. Together, we turned their needs for tissue, clinical trial networks, pristine data, and new drugs into the most innovative models the country had seen. New drugs—effective drugs—were emerging faster than we'd ever seen in the pharmaceutical industry. If we had one treatment, we needed the next one, yesterday. Patients were relapsing, dying. I ran every meeting with the same directness, and intensity, urging a very polite group of scientists to say exactly what they thought, collaborate, and not to dare accept our precious MMRF funding unless the timelines could be hit. Hiring people at the MMRF with the same fearless impatience allowed us to keep up the pace. With fifteen drugs approved, lifetimes tripled, quadrupled, and a cure on the horizon, I have lived a life of extraordinary purpose. Sharing the MMRF model and business plan with every cancer who wanted it at Harvard Business School's Kraft Accelerator was the icing on the cake. As was writing this book, the only way I knew to help all of you.

Becoming fearless allowed me to take the risks that gave our family one of its greatest gifts—David. I knew from the first pages in that sunflower journal, the importance of having Karen as a sidekick in my life. I could sense that growing up without a mom would not be an easy ride. In those early days, it was clear, I was doing IVF for Paul and Nicole. Yet every day was a new moment with our beautiful unit of four. Every day I saw something that made me quietly pray to see it again or even better, see the next thing. We were blessed to have two children who were in many ways polar opposites but loved each other so much. Nicole's boundless capacity for kindness, sensitivity, and her quiet gentle nature were balanced by David's energy, dry sense of humor, and keen ability to sense what you're thinking. And then the next risk. Who in their right mind would decide to deal with cancer, pregnancy, and a move across the country? But with two years to go, it was doable.

A counselor gave me a great piece of advice when I started heading to active disease and chemotherapy. *Don't put all of this on Paul and your sister, spread the needs to your friends. Reach out to them now and let them support you with meals, notes, humor, whatever will get you through. Tell them what scares you most when you're sad.*

I called a lunch meeting of this somewhat disparate group of seven working moms, eight including myself, who never ate lunch. I told them my disease was active and that I needed them. They picked up the ball and ran with it. What I didn't anticipate was how *the eight* would help one another through endless difficulties over the years, through alcoholism, divorce, struggling children, sick parents, menopause, you name it. When I was later diagnosed with breast cancer, we had this down. Walk it out, talk it out, make a plan.

Yes, being fearless brought me, against all odds, a cure (for me and thousands of others), a purposeful life, the most precious unit of four, a loving and hilariously funny extended family, traditions for the ages, and friendships to last a lifetime. But now, after so many things had settled, I was making up for the cost of that fearlessness. I've told you all of this because I want you to know what I didn't, to perhaps help you to avoid some heartache or if not avoid it, to know that you are not alone in it. And that there's power in asking for forgiveness.

The Final WTDs

First, apologize. I had to apologize to Paul for not seeing all he'd given up to care for me. When I started this book, I began re-creating all the "moments" along my cancer journey. His sacrifices were decades long, with the list going all the way back to the day he sold his first company twenty-five years ago.

Next, I had to apologize to Karen. Her sacrifice was extraordinary. Not only had she saved my life with her immune system, she had lived with me during that transplant and the ensuing depression, at a time when her own world was falling apart. She was separated and headed to divorce and yet the cancer card always won. Death trumped divorce, or so I thought back then. Karen understood. "Of course it was hard," she said, "but I wouldn't change any of it." Our conversation taught us that empathy is the key to seeing our way through. We're both better people as a result.

And then I apologized to Nicole. I asked her directly what she thought of me and had tears rolling down my face when she said rather haltingly, "You were so hard on me." When I asked for the details, she said, "You expected way too much. You had a vision of what you thought my life should be and you had just *that* short window to make sure I got it done." It was true—I'd always thought I had to spew it all out before that infamous relapse happened. But there was forgiveness in her words as well. She told me if one person has the gift to change the world for thousands of people, even if there will be sacrifices, they should do it.

And last there was David. "I feel like you deserve an apology from me," I told him. He was walking to work when I called, I could hear the horns honking behind him. He's happy. He's back at NBC and is planning on moving in with Abby.

"Why would I need an apology?"

"Don't you feel there were times when I wasn't there?"

"Yes, but you were sick, you were working hard. You may not have always understood exactly what I was going through, but we did talk. You did listen. I always knew how much you cared."

And there you have it. Talking matters. So does listening. These conversations were necessary and a part of my healing. They were clearly unified on one point: I was a demanding wife, mother, sister, and patient. While I was glad to know they understood, their disappointment was obvious and needed to be acknowledged.

I spoke with *the eight* as well. We never stopped talking. And when I offered an apology to my friends, their response was so them. *Kathy, we get it. We're still proud of you. You were just trying to help everyone around you. It came at a cost. We're just glad you're back.*

My second box to check in my reset was to think through who I wanted to be now. Could I change after being so demanding, so hard-edged, for so long? I wondered that, too. Until my friend Bonnie showed up on my doorstep with that big cup of coffee. Until Tiffany brought me ginger tea and shared her most vulnerable moments in her breast cancer journey. Until Bridget texted every morning to walk with me and just talk—she was the master of seeing every new flower, every prettily painted door, every precocious child.

So I did what I've always done. I let my curious mind take over. I went into research mode listening to Kate Bowler, Suleika Jaouad, Maya Shankar, Adam Grant, Brené Brown, Jon Gottman, Terry Real, Peter Attia, and Glennon Doyle podcasts on my long walks in the beautiful park near our house. And slowly, I started to laugh, appreciate the seasons, look forward to the next holiday, stick with the traditions that truly mattered.

And last, as I turn the pages to the next chapter of my life, I hope I've learned that while it's important to fear *less*, it's also important to live *more*, to stay connected to the people who matter most, the ones bending their lives for your survival. Without appropriate boundaries and care and nurturing, fearlessness can be fatal. If you or a loved one are ever facing a fatal diagnosis, remember these final three WTDs from my final (for the moment) reset:

✓ **Say thank you. Don't ever take kindness for granted.**
✓ **Speak up. Don't ever let resentment build.**
✓ **Apologize. It's never too late.**

"I love you" never hurts, either.

ACKNOWLEDGMENTS

Like most things in life, writing a book is a team effort. I did not write this book alone. I wrote it with my dearest friend and colleague who has known me for over a decade, shares my passion for healthcare, and understands the double-edged sword of my life: I'm tough and demanding because I care too much—about my fellow patients, and the family and friends I love most. Michael Schubert worked with me nearly every day, despite his own demanding job, to make sure this book resonated for as many people as possible. He was my sounding board, my confidant, my editor, and my cheerleader. I am forever grateful for his wisdom, wit, and willingness to learn right alongside me.

As Katie Couric noted in her beautifully written Foreword, we have known each other over twenty years. I swear we were sisters in a previous life but honestly, Katie has this extraordinary ability make everyone feel important, close, seen, and heard. We share one common goal—to make sure every patient has access to the best medical care; we have watched way too many people suffer. Working with such a dear friend to get this book in the hands of the people who need it most was not only important, it was fun. Everything with Katie is both important and joyful.

Lee Woodruff also encouraged me to get my story out there. We worked closely together capturing the most important events in those thirty journals stacked high on my credenza. She helped me bring them to life and create learning moments for the reader.

And to David Black, agent extraordinaire, who believed in this book from day one and personally saw it through from beginning to end. David, thank you for realizing cancer patients desperately need a playbook for their disease, that families must know their health risks and take action, and that everyone needs a hopeful story as well. Thank you, Karen Rinaldi and the entire HarperCollins team for your leadership and patience in teaching a novice like me how to get it right in the publishing field. Special thanks to Yelena Nesbit, Rachel Kambury, Jessica Gilo, and Sacha Chadwick for sharing my vision while focusing on the details, too. While writing a book is intense, so is making sure the people who need it most know it's out there. Sandi Mendelson and her amazing team at Hilsinger-Mendelson worked wisely and tirelessly to reach patients, caregivers, and people at risk of any disease.

There are three women who were instrumental in my life; they always saw the good and tolerated the not-so-great. They never wanted to be front and center and yet many of my accomplishments can be attributed to them. All three have the same important genes—those that focus on loyalty and the ability to say what they think—directly and honestly. Catherine Gallen has been beside me from the day Nicole was born. We interviewed Cat twenty-nine years ago as a nanny when she arrived from Ireland; she is still an integral part of our family today. Now a nurse practitioner, there is nothing she can't do to make our lives easier, better, happier. Shannon Powell was my executive assistant for over fifteen years. She was the master people connector, scheduling maestro, and believer. Anne Quinn Young, now chief mission officer at the MMRF, was one of our first hires at the foundation, and undoubtedly our best. She is the greatest gift to cancer patients and their families and was right beside me breaking down every barrier in our broken healthcare system.

Thank you to my beautiful family that I listed in the front of this book as FamJam. I love each and every one of you. Paul, it wasn't the life you planned for, but I couldn't have done it without you. I will never be able to thank you enough. Nicole, I started that sunflower journal saying, "You make life worth living," and you do. Every single day in every way. David, I always say, "We've never had a sad day since the day you were born" and it's true. You bring light and humor to everything you do. Karen, thank you for literally saving my life, hearing me out, and sharing our family's traditions. I think Mom would be proud of both of us. JJ, Katy, and Tyler, thank you for being "the cousins" who no matter how much the parents screw it up, will all prevail. And finally, to my dearest friends, "the eight," we could write another entire book on our lives together. We have faced many an adversity, crossed many a bridge, and created the best bucket list out there; we have laughed, cried, and lived.

Most important, thank you to the patients who show such courage, to their caregivers who sacrifice endlessly, and to the clinicians and scientist who give their lives to finding cures.

INDEX

Note: The abbreviation KG refers to Kathy Giusti.

ABOUT THE AUTHOR

KATHY GIUSTI is a two-time cancer survivor, business leader, and healthcare disrupter. Named as one of *Time* magazine's 100 Most Influential People and *Fortune* magazine's World's 50 Greatest Leaders, Giusti is recognized as a pioneer in precision medicine. She founded the Multiple Myeloma Research Foundation (MMRF), cochaired the Harvard Business School (HBS) Kraft Precision Medicine Accelerator, and has worked with three American presidents to fight and cure cancer. Kathy works to push for change where it's needed most, to fix what is broken so that everyone may heal, and to simplify the journey for others, so that they can heal themselves.